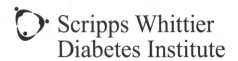

Scripps Whittier
Diabetes Institute

GUIDE TO PATIENT MANAGEMENT & PREVENTION OF DIABETES

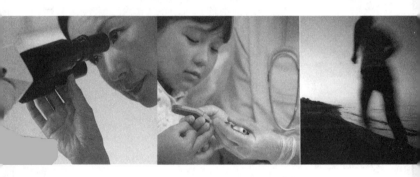

ATHENA PHILIS-TSIMIKAS, MD
Corporate Vice President
Scripps Whittier Diabetes Institute
La Jolla, California

STEPHANIE DECKER, RN, CDE
Manager of Pr_____ ___
Scripps Whitt
La Joll

D1385194

JONES AND BARTLETT PUBLISHERS
Sudbury, Massachusetts
BOSTON   TORONTO   LONDON   SINGAPORE

World Headquarters

Jones and Bartlett Publishers	Jones and Bartlett	Jones and Bartlett Publishers
40 Tall Pine Drive	Publishers Canada	International
Sudbury, MA 01776	6339 Ormindale Way	Barb House, Barb Mews
978-443-5000	Mississauga, Ontario L5V 1J2	London W6 7PA
info@jbpub.com	Canada	United Kingdom
www.jbpub.com		

Jones and Bartlett's books and products are available through most bookstores and online booksellers. To contact Jones and Bartlett Publishers directly, call 800-832-0034, fax 978-443-8000, or visit our website, www.jbpub.com.

Substantial discounts on bulk quantities of Jones and Bartlett's publications are available to corporations, professional associations, and other qualified organizations. For details and specific discount information, contact the special sales department at Jones and Bartlett via the above contact information or send an email to specialsales@jbpub.com.

Production Credits
Chief Executive Officer: Clayton Jones
Chief Operating Officer: Don W. Jones, Jr.
President, Higher Education and Professional Publishing: Robert W. Holland, Jr.
V.P., Sales: William J. Kane
V.P., Design and Production: Anne Spencer
V.P., Manufacturing and Inventory Control: Therese Connell
Executive Publisher: Christopher Davis
Senior Marketing Manager: Barb Bartoszek
Senior Acquisitions Editor: Alison Hankey
Editorial Assistant: Sara Cameron
Production Manager: Jenny L. Corriveau
Composition: diacriTech, Chennai, India
Cover Design: Kristin E. Parker
Cover and Title Page Images: (left) © Tom Grill/ShutterStock, Inc.; (middle) © Anette Romanenko/
  Dreamstime.com; (right) © Roca/ShutterStock, Inc.
Printing and Binding: Malloy, Inc.
Cover Printing: Malloy, Inc.

Library of Congress Cataloging-in-Publication Data
Philis-Tsimikas, Athena.
  Scripps Whittier Diabetes Institute guide to patient management & prevention of diabetes / Athena
  Philis-Tsimikas, Stephanie Decker.
    p. ; cm.
  Includes bibliographical references and index.
  ISBN-13: 978-0-7637-7326-7 (pbk.)
  ISBN-10: 0-7637-7326-3 (pbk.)
  1. Diabetes—Handbooks, manuals, etc. I. Decker, Stephanie. II. Scripps Whittier Diabetes Institute. III. Title.
  [DNLM: 1. Diabetes Mellitus—diagnosis—Handbooks. 2. Diabetes Mellitus—therapy—Handbooks.
  WK 39 P564s 2010]
  RC660.P465 2010
  616.4'62—dc22
                                    2009043620
6048

Printed in the United States of America
14 13 12 11 10   10 9 8 7 6 5 4 3 2 1

Contents

About the Authors

Athena Philis-Tsimikas, MD

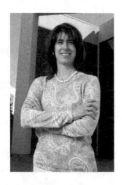

Dr. Tsimikas received her medical degree from the University of Athens Medical School, Athens, Greece in 1988. She is certified by the American Board of Internal Medicine in the subspecialty of Diabetes and Endocrinology. She served as a clinical endocrinologist on the staff of the Scripps Clinic Medical Group for 7 years from 1994 to 2001. She assisted in establishing the community-wide, nationally recognized diabetes program, Project Dulce, in 1997 and subsequently joined The Whittier Institute full-time in 2001. She was named Executive Director for the Scripps Whittier Diabetes Institute in 2004 and Corporate Vice President in May of 2008.

Stephanie Decker, RN, CDE

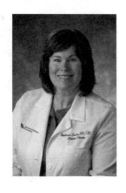

Ms. Decker is the Manager of Professional Education and Training at the Scripps Whittier Diabetes Institute, La Jolla, California. An RN, CDE for 15 years, she enjoys creating and implementing diabetes training programs for healthcare professionals throughout the United States. Her other experiences include working with low income and culturally diverse community clinics, as well as diabetes care and management in the hospital setting.

She is a member of the American Association of Diabetes Educators, is the past President of the San Diego Association of Diabetes Educators, and is a board member of the Behavioral Diabetes Institute.

Introduction

The attention on diabetes has shifted dramatically in the last 20 years. The prevalence rates of the disease have skyrocketed worldwide while the lines between the classic diagnoses of type 1 and type 2 diabetes have blurred with a rising number of children being diagnosed with "adult-onset diabetes." A plethora of innovative therapies has been introduced into the market, yet our best ammunition in the struggle against diabetes remains clear: practical, evidence-based education for clinicians and patients. Education is critical for modifying lifestyles, including behavioral approaches to preventing and controlling the disease. Training teams of physicians and nurses on how to initiate appropriate medical regimens is also important, and providing tools and approaches for preventing comorbid conditions of diabetes that lead to premature death should be a standard for ensuring best quality care.

The rates of developing diabetes continue to rise and are predicted to hit 366 million people worldwide by the year 2030. This guide offers resources that have been developed, tested, and implemented successfully in a variety of real-world, healthcare settings, including diverse, ethnic communities throughout the nation, and can be used in a productive way all over the world. Over the last 15 years, our goal at Scripps Whittier Diabetes Institute has been to develop teams of experts that work in partnership with our physicians, patients, and communities to deliver the best possible approaches to care and prevention of diabetes. Our research has demonstrated improved health, behavioral, and financial outcomes. We trust that you will find these resources useful in building your successful programs.

Athena Philis-Tsimikas, MD
Corporate Vice President
Scripps Whittier Diabetes Institute

1 ■ Epidemic of Diabetes

The Global Perspective

Every 10 seconds, two people in the world will develop diabetes.[1] It is currently estimated that 250 million people worldwide are living with diabetes. By 2025, this number is expected to increase to more than 380 million people.[2]

The regions with the highest rates are in the eastern Mediterranean and Middle East, where 9.2% of the adult population has diabetes. North America currently has a rate of 8.4%.[3] **Table 1.1** shows the current and future predicted rates of diabetes in various countries.

Global Costs of Diabetes

In poor countries, type 1 diabetes in particular is costly in terms of mortality.[4] Many children die because of an inability to obtain insulin. Premature death is a certainty for people with diabetes in many developing countries because of lack of funding and access to medical care. For example, a person in Mozambique who requires insulin will be dead in 12 months.

Diabetes affects all people in society, not just those who live with diabetes. The World Health Organization estimates the cost of treating stroke, heart disease, and mortality, as well as the loss of income due to disability in 2005 was approximately $250 billion in China, $225 billion in the Russian Federation, and $210 billion in India. If nothing is done soon to address the global epidemic and management of diabetes, government budgets will face an enormous financial strain related to persons with disabilities, decreased productivity, increased medical expenses, and lost revenue.

Table 1.1   Current and Future Diabetes Predictions

2007 PEOPLE WITH DIABETES AGES 20–79 YEARS (MILLIONS)		2025 PEOPLE WITH DIABETES AGES 20–79 YEARS (MILLIONS)	
India	40.9	India	69.9
China	39.8	China	59.3
United States	19.2	United States	25.4
Russian Federation	9.6	Brazil	17.6
Germany	7.4	Pakistan	11.5
Japan	7.0	Mexico	10.8
Pakistan	6.9	Russian Federation	10.3
Brazil	6.9	Germany	8.1
Mexico	6.1	Egypt	7.6
Egypt	4.4	Bangladesh	7.4

2007 PREVALENCE WITH DIABETES AGES 20–79 YEARS (%)		2025 PREVALENCE WITH DIABETES AGES 20–79 YEARS (%)	
Nauru	30.7	Nauru	30.7
United Arab Emirates	19.5	United Arab Emirates	19.5
Saudi Arabia	16.7	Saudi Arabia	16.7
Bahrain	15.2	Bahrain	15.2
Kuwait	14.4	Kuwait	14.4
Oman	13.1	Oman	13.1
Tonga	12.9	Tonga	12.9
Mauritius	11.1	Mauritius	11.1
Egypt	11.0	Egypt	11.0
Mexico	10.6	Mexico	10.6

Source: International Diabetes Federation. Contents: data tables. In: *IDF Diabetes Atlas*. 4th ed. Available at: http://www.eatlas.idf.org/. Accessed October 20, 2009.

The Epidemic in the United States

The following figures illustrate the diabetes epidemic in the United States[5]:

Pre-diabetes: 57 million people
Undiagnosed: 5.7 million people
Diagnosed: 17.9 million people
Total: 23.6 million children and adults

The following social and cultural changes contribute to the epidemic of diabetes both in the United States and globally:

- Poor lifestyle habits, such as inactivity, obesity, and low-quality food choices, are the primary cause of the epidemic.
- Cultural changes include:
  - Increased television and computer time
  - Frequent use of convenience and fast foods, dining out
  - Aging population
  - Economic growth that provides opportunities to purchase cars, televisions, and computers (items that contribute to sedentary lifestyles)
  - Job stress and increased work hours

Ethnic Prevalence

Age-adjusted prevalence data from the 2004–2006 National Survey are as follows[6]:

- Non-Hispanic whites: 6.6%
- Asian Americans: 7.5%
- Hispanics: 10.4%
  - Cubans: 8.2%
  - Mexican Americans: 11.9%
  - Puerto Ricans: 12.6%
- Non-Hispanic blacks: 11.8%
- Native Americans
  - Alaska Natives: 6%
  - In southern Arizona: 29.3%

U.S. Costs of Diabetes

The 2007 costs of diabetes are as follows[7]:

- *Total cost:* $174 billion
- *Direct medical costs:* $116 billion
- *Indirect costs:* $58 billion
    - 15 million sick days
    - 120 million reduced-productivity days
    - Disability (reduced productivity for those not in the labor force ($0.8 billion), unemployment from disease-related disability ($7.9 billion), and lost productive capacity due to early mortality ($26.9 billion).[8]

Personal Costs of Diabetes in the United States

The 2006 National Healthcare Disparities Report finds disparities related to ethnicity, race, and socioeconomic status still pervade in the U.S. healthcare system.[9] People living in the United States have some of the same barriers to diabetes self-care as do those in poorer countries, namely, limited access to quality health care, personal financial and health insurance limitations, and cultural beliefs related to seeking medical care.

In 2003, 5.2 million people with diabetes had a cardiovascular diagnosis, and 50,000 people with diabetes required ongoing dialysis treatments. In 2007, 873,000 people with diabetes had a primary or secondary diagnosis of lower extremity condition.[10] It is easy to see that for the patient, his or her family, and the community the personal and financial costs of diabetes and the complications of diabetes can add to the burden of living with a chronic disease.

What Can You Do?

- Educate yourself and stay informed about the current clinical management recommendations:
    - The American Diabetes Association makes its most current clinical recommendations available every January at http://professional.diabetes.org/CPR_Search.aspx.

○ The American Association of Clinical Endocrinologists is another great diabetes resource at http://www.aace.com.
- Actively work with your state government and the federal government to improve diabetes care:
  ○ The Agency for Healthcare Research and Quality has developed a resource titled "Diabetes Care Quality Improvement: A Resource Guide for State Action" that you can access at http://www.ahrq.gov/qual/diabqual/diabqguide.htm.
  ○ Join the American Diabetes Association Advocacy Center, which works on the local and federal levels. You can sign up to become a diabetes advocate at http://advocacy.diabetes.org/site/PageServer?pagename=AC_homepage.

References

1. Discovery Health. *Diabetes: A Global Epidemic Part 1*. Available at: http://discoveryhealthcme.discovery.com/beyond/miniPlayer.html?playerId=1312399220. Accessed October 20, 2009.

2. Silink M. Foreword. In: International Diabetes Federation, *IDF Diabetes Atlas*. 4th ed. Available at: http://www.eatlas.idf.org/newsc269.html. Accessed October 20, 2009.

3. International Diabetes Federation. Contents: data tables. In: *IDF Diabetes Atlas*. 4th ed. Available at: http://www.eatlas.idf.org/. Accessed October 20, 2009.

4. International Diabetes Federation. Contents: economic impacts of diabetes. In: *IDF Diabetes Atlas*. 4th ed. Available at: http://www.eatlas.idf.org/.

5. American Diabetes Association. Total prevalence of diabetes and pre-diabetes. Available at: http://www.diabetes.org/diabetes-statistics/prevalence.jsp. Accessed October 20, 2009.

6. National Diabetes Information Clearinghouse. National diabetes statistics, 2007: race and ethnic differences in the prevalence of diagnosed diabetes. Available at: http://diabetes.niddk.nih.gov/dm/pubs/statistics/#race. Accessed October 20, 2009.

7. US Department of Health and Human Services, Centers for Disease Control and Prevention. *National Diabetes Fact Sheet 2007*. Available at: http://www.cdc.gov/diabetes/pubs/pdf/ndfs_2007.pdf. Accessed October 20, 2009.

8. American Diabetes Association. Economic costs of diabetes in the U. S. in 2007. *Diabetes Care.* 2008;31:596–615.

9. US Department of Health and Human Services, Agency for Healthcare Research and Quality. *National Healthcare Disparities Report, 2006.* Available at: http://www.ahrq.gov/qual/nhdr06/nhdr06.htm. Accessed October 20, 2009.

10. US Department of Health and Human Services, Centers for Disease Control and Prevention. Number (in millions) of persons with diabetes aged 35 years and older with self-reported cardiovascular disease conditions, United States, 1997–2007. Available at: http://www.cdc.gov/diabetes/statistics/cvd/fig1.htm. Accessed October 20, 2009.

2 ▪ Classifications of Glucose Disorders[1]

Categories of Increased Risk for Diabetes: Pre-Diabetes, Impaired Fasting Glucose (IFG), Impaired Glucose Tolerance (IGT)

Screening

Fasting plasma glucose (FPG) or 2-hr 75-g oral glucose tolerance test (OGTT). An OGTT may better define the risk of diabetes in patients who have impaired fasting glucose.

Candidates for Screening

Any adult with a body mass index (BMI) greater than or equal to 25 kg/m² and who has risk factors such as the following:

- Inactivity
- First-degree relative with diabetes
- Diagnosis of gestational diabetes or delivered a baby greater than 9 lb
- High-risk ethnic group such as African American, Latino, Pacific Islander, Asian American, or Native American
- Diagnosis of hypertension or dyslipidemia
- Acanthosis nigricans noted on skin (darkening of skin on the neck or underarms, under the breasts, in the groin area)

If no risk factors are present, start screening at age 45 and repeat testing every 3 years unless you note risk factors, and then screen earlier.

Diagnosis[2]

FPG ≥100 mg/dL and <126 mg/dL or 2-hr OGTT ≥140 mg/dL and <200 mg/dL or A, C 5.7–6.4%.

Treatment

- Nutrition counseling with a focus on healthy foods and portion sizes.
- Walking or some activity at least 150 minutes per week. Patients can begin activity gradually and work up to 150 minutes per week.
- Weight loss of 5% to 10% based on the Diabetes Prevention Program study results.
- Consider metformin therapy if risk factors are present such as hypertension, dyslipidemia, obesity, primary relative with diabetes, and the patient is younger than 60 years of age.

Prevention

Early assessment of risk factors and lifestyle counseling with patient and the entire family.

Metabolic Syndrome

Metabolic syndrome is also called the insulin resistance syndrome.[3] Genetic predisposition, excess body fat, and physical inactivity all contribute to the risk of developing this cluster of disorders, all of which put the patient at risk of coronary heart disease, stroke, and other diseases related to vascular changes.

Diagnosis

You can make a diagnosis of metabolic syndrome if three or more of the following factors are present:

- Central obesity as measured by waist circumference:
  - Men—Greater than or equal to 40 inches
  - Women—Greater than or equal to 35 inches
  - Asian men—Greater than or equal to 35.4 inches[4]
  - Asian women—Greater than or equal to 31.5 inches
- Fasting blood triglycerides greater than or equal to 150 mg/dL
- High-density lipoprotein (HDL) cholesterol:
  - Men—Less than 40 mg/dL
  - Women—Less than 50 mg/dL

- Blood pressure greater than or equal to 130/85 mm Hg
- Fasting glucose greater than or equal to 100 mg/dL

Treatment

- Offer lifestyle counseling on weight loss, daily activity, healthy food choices, and portion sizes.
- Treat hypertension or dyslipidemia with medications per established guidelines.
- Assess cardiovascular and cerebral vascular risk factors.
- Discuss other habits: stopping smoking, limiting alcohol to one or two drinks daily.

Prevention

Early assessment of risk factors and lifestyle counseling with patient and entire family.

Polycystic Ovarian Syndrome

Polycystic ovarian syndrome (PCOS) may be present in up to half of all women with type 2 diabetes.[5] It affects the menstrual cycle, as well as the ability to have children, and increases the risk of coronary and vascular disease.[6] Women typically seek medical care when they are having difficulty conceiving or are concerned about their physical appearance related to elevated androgen levels.

Screening

In the absence of pregnancy and when amenorrhea or oligomenorrhea has persisted for 6 months, a careful history and examination should be done to evaluate the possible diagnosis of PCOS.[7]

Diagnosis

Clinical features of PCOS are the following[6,7]:

- Hirsutism
- Acne
- Central obesity

- Weight gain
- Mood fluctuations, depression
- Elevated testosterone level
- Elevated luteinizing hormone
- Normal to mildly elevated follicle stimulating hormone
- Hyperinsulinemia
- Follicular cysts
- Amenorrhea, oligomenorrhea
- Dyslipidemia
- Hypertension
- Male-patterned baldness
- Acanthosis nigricans
- Skin tags
- Sleep apnea

Treatment[6,7]

- Progesterone birth control pill (to control cycle, decrease androgens)
- Metformin (for insulin resistance, to decrease androgen levels)
- Clomiphene citrate (for fertility)
- Spironolactone (for hirsutism)
- Lifestyle changes, weight loss, daily activity, healthy foods and portions

Prevention

Assessment and lifestyle counseling early in childhood to prevent possible onset in teenage years especially if other female family members have PCOS.

Type 2 Diabetes

Type 2 diabetes is the most common form of diabetes, accounting for 85% to 90% of all cases of diabetes.[1] There is a genetic link that is greatly affected by lifestyle behaviors. Some obese children with a family history of type 2 diabetes develop type 2 diabetes prior to adulthood.

Screening

FPG or 2-hr 75-g OGTT. An OGTT may better define the risk of diabetes in patients who have impaired fasting glucose.

Candidates for Screening

Screen any adult with a BMI ≥25 kg/m^2 and who has risk factors such as the following:

- Inactivity
- First-degree relative with diabetes
- Diagnosis of gestational diabetes or delivered of a baby >9 lb
- High-risk ethnic group such as African American, Latino, Pacific Islander, Asian American, or Native American
- Diagnosis of hypertension or dyslipidemia
- Acanthosis nigricans noted on skin (darkening of skin on the neck or underarms, under the breasts, in the groin area)

If no risk factors are present, start screening at age 45 and repeat testing every 3 years unless risk factors are noted, and then screen earlier.

Diagnosis

FPG ≥126 mg/dL repeated on two separate occasions *or*
Random glucose ≥200 mg/dL with signs and symptoms of
    diabetes *or*
2-hr 75-g OGTT ≥200 mg/dL or A, C ≥6.5%*

Other labs you can use are as follows:

- C-peptide level to evaluate insulin production (0.5 to 2.0 ng/mL [nanograms per milliliter], normal values may vary among different laboratories).

---

* The A, C test should be performed using a method certified by the National Glycohemoglobin Standardization Program. Point of care A, C at this time should not be used to diagnose diabetes. Go to www.ngsp.org/prog/index3.html for a list of A, C assays and the effect of abnormal hemoglobins. Diagnosis of diabetes during pregnancy or iron deficiency require a lab glucose.

- Some ketones may be present in patients with prolonged hyperglycemia as a result of the breakdown of fat for energy in the absence of sufficient insulin.

Treatment

Please see Chapter 3, Medications, for detailed information.

- Lifestyle modifications and metformin at diagnosis.
- Patient may require insulin initially if glucose levels and A1c are very high.
- Diabetes education classes.

Other Considerations with Type 2 Diabetes

Hyperosmolar hyperglycemic state (HHS)[8]:

- Seen more often in older adults who live alone.
- Blood glucose (BG) >600 mg/dL with no diabetic ketoacidosis (DKA) present.
- Leading causes: New onset diabetes or an infection (60%).
- Other causes: Glucocorticoids, diuretics, pancreatitis, gastrointestinal bleed, or myocardial infarction.
- Patient may present with mental status changes or neurological signs and symptoms.
- Also seeing a higher rate of known history of diabetes coming in with HHS as a result of poor diabetes management (stopped taking medications typically).
- Higher mortality than DKA because no medical help is sought for weeks or months.
- Severe dehydration and electrolyte imbalance.
- Treat with IV fluids, insulin, and electrolyte replacement.
- Treat any underlying cause.
- Patient may or may not need insulin at time of discharge.
- Resource for HHS:
  - Kitabchi AE, Kreisberg RA, Murphy MB, Umpierrez GE. Hyperglycemic crisis in adult patients with diabetes. *Diabetes Care.* 2006;29:2739–2748.

Older adults:

- Older adults have a higher risk of hypoglycemia resulting from renal changes, comorbidities, visual acuity, dexterity and accuracy concerns with blood glucose monitoring, and, for some, memory problems.
- For patients with self-care and safety concerns, individualize A1c and glucose goals to decrease the risk of hypoglycemia. Consider an A1c between 7.0 and 7.5 vs. <7.
- Simplify medication regimens (order combination medications when possible) and remember financial constraints for those on a fixed budget when prescribing medications.
- Engage home health care, case management, and social worker as needed.
- Communicate medication changes and care with other physicians seeing the patient to avoid multiple similar disease prescriptions, which are more commonly seen in the older population.

Children with Type 2 Diabetes

Screening

Children age 10 or younger if puberty occurs earlier than age 10, with a BMI >85th percentile for age and sex, weight for height >85th percentile, or weight >120% of ideal for height and any two of the following risk factors:

- Family history of type 2 diabetes in first- or second-degree relative
- High-risk ethnic group, such as African American, Latino, Pacific Islander, Asian American, or Native American
- Acanthosis nigricans
- Hypertension
- Dyslipidemia
- PCOS

- Maternal history of diabetes or gestational diabetes during the child's gestation
- Small-for-gestational-age birthweight

FPG is the recommended screening for children. If FPG is normal, rescreen in 3 years.

- Same diagnostic criteria and labs as type 2 adult. If there is any concern that the patient has type 1 vs. type 2 diabetes, then order islet cell autoantibodies (ICA), glutamic acid decarboxylase (GAD), and insulin autoantibodies (IAA) to rule out a diagnosis of type 1 diabetes.

Treatment of Children with Type 2 Diabetes

- Lifestyle counseling: Assess parent's cultural belief system and understanding of healthy eating. Some cultures feel being overweight is a sign of success and happiness.
- Medications: Metformin and glimepiride (8 years of age or older) are currently approved by the Food and Drug Administration for use in children.[9] Insulin therapy is also an option.
- Goal is to have fasting glucose <126 mg/dL and A, C <7%.

The recommended glucose goals for children with Type I diabetes are shown in **Table 2.1.**[1]

Table 2.1   ADA Glucose Recommendations for Children and Adolescents with Type I diabetes

AGE	PRE-MEAL	BEDTIME	A1C	CAUTION
Toddlers/ preschool up to age 6 yrs	100–180 mg/dL	110–200 mg/dL	<8.5% (but >7.5%)	Risk and vulnerability for hypoglycemia
School age 6–12 yrs	90–180 mg/dL	100–180 mg/dL	<8%	Risk of hypoglycemia
Adolescents and young adults 13–19 yrs	90–130 mg/dL	90–150 mg/dL	<7.5%	Risk for severe hypoglycemia

Gestational Diabetes

Gestational diabetes (GDM) is defined as any degree of glucose intolerance first noted during pregnancy.

Screening and Diagnosis[1]

Complete screening between 24 and 28 weeks of gestation. Women at very high risk for GDM should be screened for diabetes as soon as possible after the confirmation of pregnancy. Criteria for very high risk are as follows:

- Prior history of GDM
- Previous delivery of large-for-gestation baby >9 lb
- Presence of glycosuria
- Severe obesity
- Diagnosis of PCOS
- Family history of type 2 diabetes

Glucose Tolerance Testing

1. Perform initial screening by measuring plasma or serum glucose 1 hr after a 50-g oral glucose load. If glucose >140 mg/dL, complete a 100-g OGTT on a separate day.
2. One-step approach (may be preferred in clinics with high prevalence of GDM): Perform a diagnostic 100-g OGTT in all women to be tested at 24–28 weeks.
3. The 100-g OGGT is diagnostic for GDM if two labs are abnormal:

Fasting: ≥95 mg/dL
1 hr: ≥180 mg/dL
2 hr: ≥155 mg/dL
3 hr: ≥140 mg/dL

Treatment

- Consultation with a registered dietitian to discuss healthy eating and caloric and nutrient needs
- Avoidance of concentrated sweets, juices, and soda, and limitation of no more than two caffeine products a day
- Walking for 15 minutes at a normal pace after each meal

- Medications: Insulin, glyburide, metformin (PCOS)
- Check BG fasting, less than 95 mg/dL, 1 hr after each main meal, <140 mg/dL[10]

Postpartum Follow-Up

- Encourage breastfeeding.
- At 6 weeks, repeat 2-hr 75-g OGTT to screen for diabetes. Five percent to 10% of women are found to have diabetes.[11]
- Women who had GDM have a 40% to 60% chance of developing type 2 diabetes in the next 5 to 10 years.[11]
- Offer lifestyle counseling to maintain healthy weight and daily activity.
- Encourage yearly lipid and glucose testing.
- Offer pre-conception planning. Women should be assessed for glucose abnormalities before trying to conceive.

Type 1 Diabetes

Type 1 diabetes accounts for 5% to 10% of all diabetes. Typically thought to occur in children only, it may occur at any age; however, the majority of people with type 1 diabetes are diagnosed younger than age 18. There is a genetic link as well as increased risk in families with autoimmune diseases.

Screening

Not recommended to screen at this time without patient exhibiting signs and symptoms.

Diagnosis

- FPG ≥126 mg/dL repeated on two separate occasions
- Random glucose ≥200 mg/dL with signs and symptoms of diabetes *or* 2-hr 75-g OGTT ≥200 mg/dL
- A, C ≥6.5%
- ICA, GAD, and IAA; one or more autoantibodies present

Other Labs

- C-peptide level to evaluate insulin production (0.5 to 2.0 ng/mL, normal values may vary among different laboratories)
- Ketones present in blood and urine
- Thyroid, thyroid-stimulating hormone, and autoantibodies[12]
- Celiac disease workup if gastrointestinal complaints. Consider serum anti-tissue transglutaminase antibodies or anti-endomysium antibodies[13]

Treatment

Please see Chapter 3 for detailed information.

- Basal and bolus insulin, injection (syringe or insulin pens), insulin pump
- Carbohydrate and correction scale counting if patient is capable of learning this treatment method
- Diabetes education classes

Other Considerations with Type 1 Diabetes

Honeymoon phase with new diagnosis of type 1 diabetes:

- Less common in young children and seen more often in older teenagers and adults, the honeymoon phase is a result of some continued beta cell function in the pancreas. The pancreas may produce small amounts of insulin for a few weeks, months, or up to a year after the diagnosis of type 1 diabetes. In this stage, less basal or bolus insulin may be required. Frequent monitoring and hypoglycemia precautions are essential. Insulin doses may significantly increase as the patient leaves the honeymoon phase.

Diabetic Ketoacidosis

Diabetic ketoacidosis (DKA) is often seen on diagnosis and may occur any time the patient has insufficient insulin doses. Some people are more prone to DKA, while others can sustain glucose levels 300 mg/dL to 400 mg/dL and not go into DKA. DKA may occur within 6 hr (insulin pump occludes) or up to 12–24 hr if taking insulin injections.

The causes of DKA are as follows:

- New diagnosis of type 1 diabetes
- Infection or severe illness, myocardial infarction, stroke, pancreatitis, trauma
- Insulin deficiency (financial, psychosocial, expired or damaged insulin—too hot or too cold temperatures)
- Severe stress

Lab Values[14]

- Glucose level ≥250 mg/dL
- Serum beta-hydroxybutyrate or urine ketones high

Treatment

- IV fluids, electrolyte replacement, and insulin drip
- Assessment and treatment of cause of DKA
- Social worker if related to psychosocial issues

Patient Education

- Causes of DKA
- Check ketones at home with urine keto-dipsticks or Precision Extra meter (measures serum ketones) if ill, very stressed, signs and symptoms of DKA are present, or glucose is ≥250 mg/dL several times
- Signs and symptoms may include nausea, vomiting, diarrhea, abdominal pain, muscle pain, fruity/acetone breath, hypotension, tachycardia, possible change in mental status
- Resource for DKA:
  - ○ Kitabchi AE, Kreisberg RA, Murphy MB, Umpierrez GE. Hyperglycemic crisis in adult patients with diabetes. *Diabetes Care*. 2006;29:2739–2748.

Other Causes of Glucose Disorders[15]

- Maturity-onset diabetes of the young:
    - Onset is before age 25 years usually.
    - Impaired insulin secretion with minimal or no defects in insulin action.
    - Autosomal dominant pattern with abnormalities at six genetic loci on different chromosomes have been identified.
    - Treatment is dependent upon glucose levels, diet and exercise, oral agents, or insulin.
- Latent autoimmune diabetes of adults[16]:
    - Typically at age 35 yrs or older.
    - Nonobese.
    - Present without ketoacidosis.
    - Hard to diagnosis at onset because of a lack of signs and symptoms. Warrants checking ICA, IAA, GAD antibodies if patient is nonobese.
    - Typically diagnosed as autoimmune beta cell destruction accelerates and patient goes into DKA.
    - Patient will eventually need insulin therapy.
- Medications:
    - Glucocorticoids
    - Nicotinic acid
    - Pentamidine
    - Vacor
    - Thyroid hormone
    - Dilantin (phenytoin)
    - Beta-adrenergic agonists
    - Alpha-interferon
    - Some antipsychotics
- Diseases of the pancreas:
    - Pancreatitis
    - Cystic fibrosis
    - Hemochromatosis
    - Neoplasm

- Endocrinopathies:
  - Hyperthyroidism
  - Cushing's syndrome
  - Pheochromocytoma
  - Somatostatinoma
  - Acromegaly
- Genetic syndromes sometimes associated with diabetes:
  - Prader-Willi syndrome
  - Huntington's chorea
  - Klinefelter's syndrome
  - Turner's syndrome
  - Down syndrome
  - Myotonic dystrophy

Web Resources

Children with Diabetes: www.childrenwithdiabetes.com

Diabetes Mall: Education, books, products, English and Spanish: www.diabetesnet.com

National Alliance for Hispanic Health: An organization focusing on improving the health and well-being of Hispanics: www.hispanichealth.org

National Black Women's Health Project (NBWHP): Black Women's Health Imperative, the new name of the NBWHP, is a leading African American health education, research, advocacy, and leadership development institution: www.blackwomenshealth.org

National Diabetes Education Initiative: Patient education brochures (English and Spanish). Medicare's Blood Sugar Testing Coverage campaign: www.ndei.org

National Diabetes Education Program (NDEP): A partnership of the National Institutes of Health, the Centers for Disease Control and Prevention, and more than 200 public and private organizations: www.ndep.nih.gov

National Institute of Diabetes and Digestive and Kidney Diseases National Diabetes Clearinghouse: A resource for educators and people with diabetes. Offers free information on diabetes topics in both English and Spanish: www.niddk.nih.gov

Taking Control of Your Diabetes (TCOYD): Diabetes education, national seminars for people with diabetes: www.tcoyd.org

Diabetes Resource Toolkit

Patient Education

2–1 Facts About Diabetes

2–2 Glucose Metabolism

2–3 Project Dulce: Types of Diabetes

2–4 Types of Diabetes

2–5 Symptoms of Diabetes

2–6 Blood Glucose Balance

2–7 Blood Glucose Levels

2–8 Estimated Average Glucose or Hemoglobin A1c (A1c)

2–9 Blood Sugar Levels and Target Numbers

2–10 Taking Care of Yourself After Having Gestational Diabetes

2–11 Healthy Eating Guidelines After Gestational Diabetes

2–12 Standards of Care

Clinical Resource

2–13 Diabetes Flow Sheet

2–1 FACTS ABOUT DIABETES

DIABETES EXPLAINED

Diabetes is a chronic disease that can be controlled but not cured. The exact cause of diabetes is not known.

Diabetes involves the functioning of the pancreas, an organ located near the stomach. When we eat food, it is broken down into sugar (also called glucose). Insulin, made by the pancreas, moves glucose (sugar) inside the body cells so it can be used for energy.

With diabetes, the body is not able to use glucose in the normal way. Either the body 1) makes very little or no insulin for its needs or 2) is unable to use insulin in the normal way. Without enough insulin, the body cannot use glucose for energy. Glucose starts building up in the bloodstream because it cannot get inside the cells. The extra glucose in the bloodstream upsets normal body functions, which can result in serious symptoms and illness, sometimes requiring hospitalization. When the blood glucose remains high for prolonged periods, it may damage the organs, even if there are no symptoms.

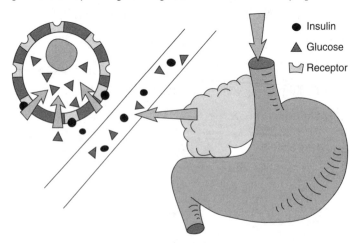

● Insulin
▲ Glucose
〰 Receptor

Insulin binds to receptors on target cells throughout the body. Only when the receptors are bound can glucose move inside the body's cells.

2–2 GLUCOSE METABOLISM

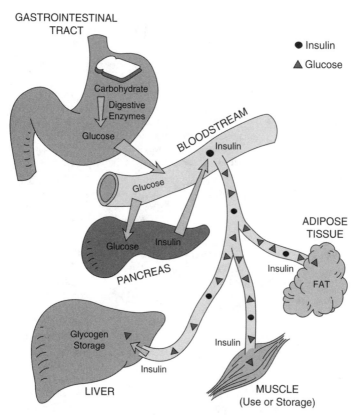

Source: Krall, L., & Beaser, R. (1989). Joslin Diabetes Manual (p. 9). Philadelphia: Lea & Febiger.

Carbohydrate is the primary source of energy for the body. The body gets its carbohydrate fuel from sugars and starches. These are digested in the gastrointestinal tract into simple sugars (example: glucose), which pass into the bloodstream. Glucose in the bloodstream stimulates the pancreas to secrete insulin. Insulin moves the glucose to muscle for use or storage, to the liver for storage as glycogen, or to adipose tissue for storage as fat.

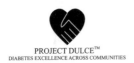

PROJECT DULCE™
DIABETES EXCELLENCE ACROSS COMMUNITIES

2–3 TYPES OF DIABETES

	TYPE 1	TYPE 2	GESTATIONAL
PHYSIOLOGICAL CAUSES	Exact cause unknown (possible causes include: injury to beta cells or virus)	Insulin resistance and/or insulin deficiency	Hormones of pregnancy cause insulin resistance
BODY TYPE	Generally thin or athletic build	Abdominal obesity; 80% are overweight	Pregnant, often pregnancy overweight
ONSET OF SYMPTOMS	Rapid onset, days to weeks in children and weeks to months in adults	Slower onset; weeks to months	Usually occurs after the 26th week of pregnancy. Related to a rise in placental hormones
TREATMENT	Insulin therapy, healthy eating patterns, and physical activity	Meal planning, regular physical activity, diabetes pills, and/or insulin therapy	Meal planning, physical activity, and/or diabetes pills or insulin therapy

2–4 TYPES OF DIABETES

Type 1 Diabetes—Insulin-Dependent Diabetes

Occurs most often in children and young adults. However, it can occur at any age. In type 1 diabetes, the pancreas stops making insulin or makes only a tiny amount. Without insulin, the body starts using fat for energy, producing harmful by-products called ketones. Insulin is necessary to life, so the hormone must be given every day.

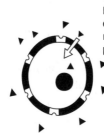

TYPE 1 DIABETES:
People with Type 1 diabetes have enough receptors, but they can't produce enough insulin.

Type 2 Diabetes

This form of diabetes generally occurs in adults, but is on the rise in children. Risk factors include family history, being overweight, a sedentary lifestyle, having diabetes during pregnancy, and being

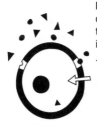

TYPE 2 DIABETES:
Most people with Type 2 diabetes either have too little insulin or are insulin resistant.

a member of certain racial or ethnic groups. African Americans, Hispanic/Latino Americans, Native Americans, and some Asian Americans and Pacific Islanders are at greater risk for type 2 diabetes.

Type 2 diabetes is the most common form of diabetes. It usually begins as insulin resistance, a disorder in which the cells in the body cannot use insulin effectively. As a result of this resistance, glucose cannot get into the body's cells and remains trapped in the bloodstream. When the blood glucose remains high, the pancreas overcompensates and produces more insulin. Eventually, the insulin-producing cells no longer function properly, resulting in decreased insulin production and elevated blood glucose levels. Type 2 diabetes is diagnosed when the fasting blood glucose is at or above 126 mg/dL or a random blood glucose is at or above 200 mg/dL or A, C ≥6.5%.

Pre-Diabetes

Pre-diabetes is a condition where the blood glucose is higher than normal, but the person does not yet have diabetes. Pre-diabetes is also called Impaired Glucose Tolerance (IGT). Studies have shown that most people with this condition develop diabetes within 10 years. Diabetes may be prevented by maintaining a healthy diet, getting regular exercise, and maintaining a healthy weight. Pre-diabetes is diagnosed with the fasting blood glucose between 100 and 125 mg/dL.

Gestational Diabetes

Some women develop diabetes during pregnancy. It usually goes away following the birth of the baby. Risk factor for future development of type 2 diabetes is approximately 50–60%.

Secondary Diabetes

This type of diabetes is caused by medications such as prednisone or some anti-psychotics, as well as diseases like Cushing's syndrome, cystic fibrosis, or pancreatitis.

Scripps Whittier
Diabetes Institute

2–5 SYMPTOMS OF DIABETES*

- Excessive thirst
- Extreme hunger
- Weight loss
- Feeling weak or tired
- Blurring of vision
- Frequent urination
- Itching, often in genital area
- Frequent yeast infections
- Changes in blood vessels (example: in the back of the eyes and lower legs)

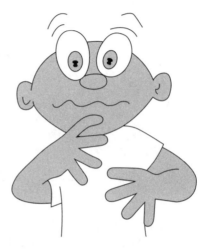

- Tingling or numbness in the legs or feet
- Skin infections or slow healing wounds (example: sores)

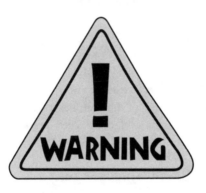

Many people have no symptoms when their blood glucose is high. It is important to test your blood glucose regularly.

2–6 Blood Glucose Balance

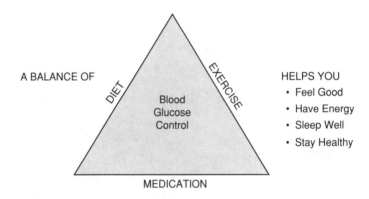

A BALANCE OF

DIET · EXERCISE · MEDICATION

Blood Glucose Control

HELPS YOU
- Feel Good
- Have Energy
- Sleep Well
- Stay Healthy

It is important for people with diabetes to keep their blood glucose levels as close to normal as possible. This may be achieved by maintaining a balance between food, exercise, and medication (if required). Research has shown that problems from diabetes can be greatly reduced by keeping the blood glucose within target ranges.

Why Control Diabetes?

The latest research conclusively proves that keeping blood glucose as close to normal as possible greatly decreases the complications of diabetes. High blood glucose, over time, can damage small blood vessels—including those of the eyes, nerves, and kidneys. Studies have shown that keeping blood glucose levels closer to normal reduces complications to small vessels by 25% to 75%.

Evaluating Blood Glucose Control

Methods to determine blood glucose control include:

Self-Monitoring Blood Glucose (SMBG) Checking blood glucose can be done by using a glucose meter (monitor). Normally, blood glucose levels will vary throughout the day from 70 to 140 mg/dL.

Scripps Whittier Diabetes Institute

Estimated Average Glucose or the Hemoglobin A1c (A1c)
This blood glucose test indicates how well diabetes has been controlled over the past 2 to 3 months. This is a blood test. The goal is <7%, which is <154 mg/dL per a glucose meter.

Urine Ketones If required, your urine can be checked as needed. Ketones in the urine means your body is using fat for energy, indicating a change is needed in your insulin regimen. Your doctor or healthcare team will explain more if ketone testing is needed.

2–7 BLOOD GLUCOSE LEVELS

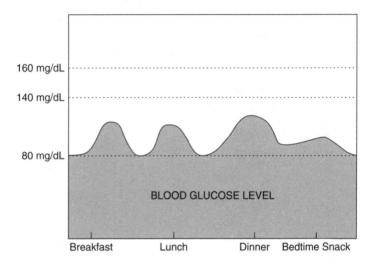

- Normally, blood glucose levels will vary throughout the day from 70 to 140 mg/dL.
- Blood glucose rises following meals and returns to pre-meal levels about 3 hours after the meal.
- To prevent high blood glucose following meals, people with diabetes should:
  - ○ Eat well-balanced meals
  - ○ Take medication on time
  - ○ Get regular exercise
  - ○ Maintain a reasonable weight

2–8 ESTIMATED AVERAGE GLUCOSE OR HEMOGLOBIN A1c (A1c)

The estimated average glucose or A1c blood glucose test indicates how well diabetes has been controlled over the past 2 to 3 months. This test is done with your lab work.

What the Numbers Mean*

Your Doctor's A1c Report	6%	7%	8%	9%	10%	11%	12%
Average Blood Glucose Range, similar to your glucose meter readings	126	154	183	212	240	269	298

Note: Standard values may vary depending on the laboratory conducting the tests; values reflected in the table should be adjusted accordingly.

2–9 BLOOD SUGAR LEVELS AND TARGET NUMBERS

Pre-Diabetes	100–125 mg/dL A, C 5.7–6.4%
Diagnosis of Diabetes	126 mg/dL or above fasting on two separate tests
	or
	200 mg/dL or above on random test with the presence of symptoms of diabetes or A, C ≥6.5%

Target Levels*

Fasting	70–130 mg/dL
2 hr. after the first bite of a meal	Below 180 mg/dL
At bedtime	100–140 mg/dL
Hypoglycemia (low blood sugar)	Below 70 mg/dL
Hyperglycemia (high blood sugar)	Above 180 mg/dL

*Note: Based on the American Diabetes Association's Clinical Practice Recommendations 2009. Your diabetes team may individualize these target numbers.

Scripps Whittier Diabetes Institute

2–10 TAKING CARE OF YOURSELF AFTER HAVING GESTATIONAL DIABETES

Here is some information for you to help you stay healthy after having gestational diabetes.

Gestational diabetes usually goes away after the birth of your baby. To be sure your blood glucose levels are returning to normal, it is recommended to check your blood glucose twice a day for the first week after delivery. Please check a fasting blood glucose and 2 hours after dinner. For an adult who is not pregnant, the normal fasting blood glucose level should be less than 100 mg/dL, and 2 hours after a meal the blood glucose should be less than 140 mg/dL. If the blood glucose level is not within the normal ranges, notify your doctor.

You should also have a 2-hour glucose tolerance test done 6 weeks after delivery by your physician to verify that you do not have diabetes. It is also recommended that you have a fasting blood glucose test, a cholesterol blood test, and a triglyceride blood test done every year at your doctor's office. Diabetes is a silent disease; the only way to know if you have it is to have a blood test.

In the future, if you decide to have another baby, you should see your doctor first. It is important to make sure your blood glucose levels are normal *before* you try to conceive. High blood glucose levels can be extremely harmful to the development of the baby in the first trimester.

A woman who has had gestational diabetes has a 50–60% chance of developing diabetes in the future. Certain ethnic populations may have a higher incidence.

The good news is, studies have shown that eating healthy, walking 30 minutes a day, and maintaining a healthy weight decrease your risk of developing diabetes. The closer you are to a healthy weight, the lower your risk is of developing diabetes.

2–11 HEALTHY EATING GUIDELINES AFTER GESTATIONAL DIABETES

- If you are planning to breast-feed, follow the same meal plan that you used while you were pregnant. Breastfeeding burns up a lot of calories and may also lower your blood glucose. If you have diabetes, talk with your physician if your blood sugar is 70 mg/dL or lower because you may need to take less of your diabetes medication.
- Try to eat balanced meals and healthy portions. Eat a snack, like a piece of fruit, if there is more than 5 hours from one meal to the next.
- Remember that fats have twice the calories of other foods, so if you need to lose weight, eat as little as possible in the fat group.
- Sweets, desserts, and sweetened beverages contain a lot of calories and very few nutrients, so eat/drink as little as possible.
- Vegetables have very few calories and help fill you up, so eat plenty.
- 1% or fat-free milks have less calories and fat.
- Avoid high-fat meats such as bacon, hotdogs, salami, pepperoni, and chorizo.
- Eating healthy and daily exercise are important for the entire family!

Summary: Are you experiencing a hard time adjusting to motherhood? Do you find yourself feeling overwhelmed, anxious, or excessively tearful? Do you feel isolated, or are you noticing concerning changes in your sleeping or eating patterns? Motherhood can be overwhelming at times. If you are having any of these feelings, please seek help from your physician.

Scripps Whittier
Diabetes Institute

2–12 STANDARDS OF CARE

Know Your Numbers

Use the following section to monitor your health and diabetes control. Know your numbers and if you do not, ask your doctor or diabetes healthcare worker.

Standards of Care for Adults with Diabetes

These standards are set by the American Diabetes Association.

TEST TO BE DONE	MONITORS	FREQUENCY OF TEST	RECOMMENDED GOALS FOR CONTROL	YOUR LAST TEST RESULTS
Estimated average glucose (doctor may say A1c)	2- to 3-month blood glucose average	Every 3 to 6 months*	<154 mg/dL (7%A1c)	
Blood pressure	Pressure within blood vessels	Every visit	<130/80 mm Hg	
Microalbumin (Urine test)	Kidney function	Yearly	Normal Range Negative or ratio below 30 mg/dL	
Creatinine (Blood test)	Kidney function	Yearly	Normal Range 0.5 to 1.2 mg/dL	
Lipid Profile Cholesterol Triglycerides HDL LDL	Risk of heart disease	Yearly with low-risk lipid values; repeat every 2 years	Chol <200 mg/dL Trig <150 mg/dL HDL: Men >40 mg/dL Women >50 mg/dL LDL <100 mg/dL	
Eye Exam- dilated	Eye disease	Yearly	Normal	

*Note: A1c test may be done at least two times a year if you are meeting treatment goals and have stable blood glucose control. We strongly encourage those with type 1 diabetes to have this test done every 3 months.

▷ Scripps Whittier Diabetes Institute

2–13 DIABETES FLOW SHEET

Name: **Medical Record #:**   **D.O.B:**

Date:					
Basic Guidelines for Diabetes Care					
Review Self-Glucose Monitoring Results (every visit)					
Blood Pressure (every visit) **Target:**					
Weight (every visit) / BMI (every visit) **Target:**					
Foot Exam (every visit)					
Dental Exam (twice per year)					
Dilated Eye Exam (yearly)					
A1C (every 3 months) Lab Range: _____ **Target:**					
Microalbuminuria (albumin/creatinine ratio)(yearly if urine protein negative)					
Estimated Glomerular Filtration Rate (GFR) (whenever chemistries are checked)					
Cholesterol (yearly) / Triglycerides (yearly) **Target:**					
HDL (yearly) / LDL (yearly) **Target:**					

Page 1 of 2. This product is part of the ***Basic Guidelines for Diabetes Care Packet*** and may be reproduced with the citation:
"Developed by the Diabetes Coalition of California and the California Diabetes Program, 2006-07."
For further information: www.caldiabetes.org or (916) 552-9888.

Influenza (yearly) / Pneumococcal Immunization (as recommended by CDC)						
Review Diabetes Health Record (DHR) (every visit)						
Self-Management Training						
Behavioral Issues / Depression						
Smoking Cessation (California Smokers' Helpline 1-800-NO-BUTTS)						
Self-Glucose Monitoring / Problem-Solving Skills						
Medication Review						
Nutrition / Weight Management						
Physical Activity						
Sick Day Management						
Hypoglycemia/ Hyperglycemia						
Foot Care						
Aspirin Therapy						
Preconception Care						
General Care						
Periodic H&P / Pap or Prostate Exam						
Mammogram / Chest X-Ray						
Screen for Colorectal Cancer						
PPD / Tetanus						
EKG						

References

1. American Diabetes Association. Standards of medical care in diabetes 2010. *Diabetes Care.* January 2010;33:s11–s61.

2. American Diabetes Association. Frequently asked questions about pre-diabetes. Available at: http://www.diabetes.org/diabetes-basics/ prevention/pre-diabetes/pre-diabetes-faqs.html. Accessed December 4, 2009.

3. American Heart Association. Metabolic syndrome: information for professionals. Available at: http://www.americanheart.org/presenter .jhtml?identifier=534%20. Accessed October 26, 2009.

4. Chan J. The metabolic syndrome: an Asian perspective. *Diabetes Voice.* May 2006;51:18–20. Available at: http://www.diabetesvoice.org/files/ attachments/article_411_en.pdf. Accessed October 26, 2009.

5. Carlsen SM, Salvesen KA, Vanky E, Fougner KJ. Polycystic ovarian syndrome and diabetes. *Tidsskr Nor Laegeforen.* October 6, 2005;125:2619–2621. Available at: http://www.ncbi.nlm.nih.gov/ pubmed/16215603. Accessed October 26, 2009.

6. US Department of Health and Human Services, Office on Women's Health, National Women's Health Information Center. Polycystic ovary syndrome (PCOS): frequently asked questions. Available at: http://www.womenshealth.gov/faq/polycystic-ovary-syndrome .cfm#i. Accessed October 26, 2009.

7. Hunter MH, Sterrett JJ. Polycystic ovary syndrome: it's not just infertility. *Am Fam Physician.* September 1, 2000;62:1079–1088, 1090.

8. American Association of Diabetes Educators. *The Art and Science of Diabetes Self-Management Education: A Desk Reference for Healthcare Professionals.* Chicago: American Association of Diabetes Educators; 2006.

9. National Diabetes Education Program. An overview of diabetes in children and adolescents, treatment strategies. Available at: http:// ndep.nih.gov/media/diabetes/youth/youth_FS.htm. Accessed October 26, 2009.

10. 2010 ADA Standards of Care. *Diabetes Care.* January 2010; 33(suppl 1):S-23.

11. National Diabetes Information Clearinghouse. National diabetes statistics, 2007. Available at: http://diabetes.niddk.nih.gov/DM/PUBS/ statistics/. Accessed October 26, 2009.

12. Pearce SHP, Merriman TR. Genetics of type I diabetes and autoimmune thyroid disease. *Endocrinol Metab Clin North Am.* June 2009;38:289–301.

13. National Diabetes Information Clearinghouse. Celiac disease. Available at: http://digestive.niddk.nih.gov/ddiseases/pubs/celiac/. Accessed October 26, 2009.

14. Trachtenberg DE. Diabetic ketoacidosis. *Am Fam Physician.* May 1, 2005;71:1705–1714.

15. American Diabetes Association. Diagnosis and classification of diabetes mellitus 2010. *Diabetes Care.* 2010;33:s65.

16. Palmer JP, Hirsch IB. What's in a name: latent autoimmune diabetes of adults, type 1.5, adult onset, and type I diabetes. *Diabetes Care.* 2003;26:536–538.

3 ▪ Medications

Primary Objective

The primary objective is to achieve healthy glucose goals in a safe manner in consideration of the patient's financial abilities, physical/mental capabilities, and support.

In the past "diet and exercise" reigned as the initial treatment of choice with slow implementation and adjustment of oral medications over a number of years. For many patients, this resulted in the development of microvascular complications. The paradigm has shifted for the better and consistent evaluation of A1c results followed by regular medication adjustment and advancement as needed is the standard of care.

Considerations for Medication Therapy

Although an A1c of <7% is generally the goal to decrease the risk of microvascular complications, individualized patient goals need to be identified using clinical judgment based on patient life expectancy, risk of hypoglycemia, cardiovascular disease, other comorbidities, and potential risks vs. benefits.[1]

Oral Agents
Which Oral Medication Treatment?

The oral antidiabetic agents are to be used with patients who have type 2 diabetes only.

1. Determine liver and renal function. Abnormal values restrict the use of some oral agents and increase the risk of hypoglycemia with sulfonylureas.
2. Do a blood glucose evaluation, A1c, fasting or random glucose. Is the patient glucose toxic? If the patient has been in a hyperglycemic state for months, typically fasting glucose is 250 mg/dL or higher, A1c is in the double digits, there is possible weight loss, or mild ketones are present. The patient

might require basal/bolus therapy initially until the patient is no longer glucose toxic (typically a few weeks), at which point oral agents would be effective.[2]

3. Does the patient have congestive heart failure (CHF) or severe cardiac disease? If yes, thiazolidinediones (TZDs) may be contraindicated and caution should be taken with metformin.

4. Consider patient education and literacy level and ability to follow through with multiple medications or dosing times. Consider combination medications and a simple medication regimen.

5. Consider the patient's ability to pay for medications. See **Table 3.1** for general pricing comparisons. Generics and older medications may need to be used. **Table 3.2** lists many oral medications and their dosages.

Biguanide[3]

Use

Primary focus is to decrease hepatic glucose dumping with secondary effect of decreasing insulin resistance.

Dosage

Starting dose of 500 mg at breakfast and at dinner. May have less chance of gastrointestinal (GI) side effects by starting with 500 mg at dinner for 1 week, and then 500 mg BID for 2 weeks. Do not increase by more than 500 mg a week to limit GI complaints. Maximum efficacy is 2000 mg/day.

Possible Side Effects

GI complaints, nausea, diarrhea, bloating, metallic taste, and flatulence are the most common and typically decrease within 2 weeks.

Precautions/Contraindications

Not to be used if glomerular filtration rate (GFR) <30 or SrCr >1.5 mg/dL in men and >1.4 mg/dL in women or liver enzymes >2.5 times normal due to risk of lactic acidosis.

Table 3.1 Oral Medication Considerations

Considerations for Use	Metformin ADA*	Sulfonylurea	TZD	DPP-4	AGI	Meglitinides
Renal issues GFR <30 Serum creatinine ♂ >1.5 mg/dL ♀ >1.4 mg/dL	do not use	caution ↑ risk of hypoglycemia	ok	Ok, dose adjustments	No studies with Cr >2	caution ↑ risk of hypoglycemia
Possible ↑ CHF	caution		do not use			
Liver ALT >2.5×†	do not use	caution	do not use	caution		caution
Insulin resistance	effective		effective			effective
Insulin deficiency		effective				maybe
Weight gain		yes	yes			
GI disturbances	yes				yes	
Possible ↑ risk bone fractures			yes			
Post-meal glucose ↓		yes		yes	yes	yes
A1c % drop‡	1–2	1–2	0.5–1.4	0.5–0.8	0.5–0.8	0.5–1.5
Cost§	$32	$20	$203	$195	$103	$175

*ADA recommends starting at onset of diagnosis of type 2 diabetes.
† No data to support use of any oral agent with severe liver disease with Child-Pugh score of 9.
‡ From: *Diabetes Care.* 2009;32:193–203.
§ From: Drugstore.com; March 2009. Prices will vary at individual locations and pharmacies.

Table 3.2   Oral Medication Names and Dosages

Generic Name*	Brand Name	Dosages / Max Dosage	Best Time
Tolazamide	Tolinase	100, 200, & 500 mg **1000 mg**	Before meals
Tolbutamide	Orinase	500 mg **3000 mg**	Before meals
Chlorpropamide	Diabinese	250 mg **750 mg**	Before meals, may last 72 hours— caution with elderly, renal
Glyburide	Diabeta	1.25, 2.5, & 5 mg **20 mg**	Either on an empty stomach or with food
	Micronase	2.5 & 5 mg **20 mg**	give BID >15 mg
	Glynase PresTab	1.5, 3, & 6 mg **12 mg**	give BID >6 mg
Glipizide	Glucotrol	5 & 10 mg **40 mg**	Take ½ hour before meal
	Glucotrol XL	2.5, 5, & 10 mg **20 mg**	Don't cut pill, time released
Glimepiride	Amaryl	1, 2, & 4 mg **8 mg**	With meals or before meal
Repaglinide	Prandin	0.5, 1, & 2 mg **16 mg**	Take 15–30 min before meal
Nateglinide	Starlix	60 & 120 mg **360 mg**	Take immediately before meals
Metformin	Glucophage	500, 850, & 1,000 mg **2,550 mg**	With meals

	Glucophage XR	500 / **2,000 mg**	Don't cut pill, time released
	Riomet	500 mg/5 mL, / 850 mg/8.5 mL / **2,550 mg/ 25.5 mL**	
Acarbose	Precose	25, 50, & 100 mg / **300 mg**	With first bite of food
Miglitol	Glyset	25, 50, & 100 mg / **300 mg**	With first bite of food
Rosiglitazone	Avandia	2, 4, & 8 mg / **8 mg**	With or without food
Pioglitazone	Actos	15, 30, & 45 mg / **45 mg**	With or without food
Sitagliptin	Januvia	25.50, & 100 mg / **100 mg**	With or without food
Saxagliptin	Onglyza	5 mg or 2.5 mg	With or without food

COMBINATION MEDICATIONS	DOSAGE
Actoplus Met = Metformin + Pioglitazone	15/500, 15/850 daily to BID
Avandamet = Metformin + Rosiglitazone	2/500, 4/500, 2/1,000, 4/1,000 daily to BID
Avandaryl = Rosiglitazone + Glimepiride	4/1, 4/2, 4/4, 8/2, 8/4, max daily dose 8/4
Duetact = Pioglitazone + Glimepiride	30/2, 30/4 once daily either dose
Glucovance = Metformin + Glyburide	1.25/250, 2.5/500, 5/500 max daily 20/2,000
Janumet = Metformin + Januvia	50/500, 50/1,000, BID
Metaglip = Metformin + Pioglitazone	2.5/250, 2.5/500, 5/500 max daily 20/2,000
PrandiMet = Prandin + Metformin	1/500, 2/500 max daily dose 10/2,500

Scripps Whittier Diabetes Institute Type 2 Patient Manual. La Jolla, Calif: Scripps Whittier Diabetes Institute; 2009.

Contraindicated with binge drinking or more than two alcoholic drinks per day. Caution with adult older than age 80 due to renal concerns and also caution with heart failure requiring pharmacological therapy. Hold if patient is in metabolic acidosis, dehydrated, NPO, or going for iodine radio contrast studies. Check liver function test once yearly. Patients with irritable bowel syndrome or any chronic bowel disorder may not be good candidates for this medication. May interfere with B_{12} and absorption, but anemia is rare.

Patient Education

1. Take regularly as prescribed because medication takes 1 month to reach effectiveness.
2. "Gas cap" for the liver (gas tank for sugar). Helps the liver to stop dumping glucose into the circulation.
3. Take with food to decrease risk of GI side effects.
4. Avoid drinking more than two alcoholic beverages a day.
5. Stop medication on the day of surgery or iodine radio contrast studies.
6. Hold if unable to drink fluids or eat due to illness (dehydration).
7. Call if unable to take medication as prescribed due to side effects, and notify an MD.
8. May cause ovulation in women with polycystic ovarian syndrome; discuss birth control and family planning options with an MD.
9. Carry ID with you that states "I have diabetes" and include MD name and phone number as well as family contact and medications.

Sulfonylureas[4]

Use

Stimulate the beta cells in the pancreas to produce insulin. These agents are effective only if the pancreas is still able to produce a sufficient amount of insulin.

Dosage

See **Table 3.2**. The risk of hypoglycemia is greatest during the first few days to 4 months when starting a sulfonylurea. Monitoring glucose levels and refraining from alcohol initially are recommended. Little benefit is noted past half of the maximum recommended dosage.

Possible Side Effects

Hypoglycemia is the biggest possible side effect. Patient education and reinforcement of how to properly take the medication are very important. Weight gain, GI complaints, headache, or sun sensitivity may occur.

Precautions/Contraindications[5]

Use in patients who have renal insufficiency or liver disease is cautioned because of increased risk of hypoglycemia and metabolism of these medications. Caution with use in older adults; patients who are debilitated, malnourished, or with inconsistent or poor food intake, as well as those with adrenal or pituitary insufficiency because of the risk of hypoglycemia. Precaution with use in patients who drink more than two alcoholic drinks a day secondary to hypoglycemia. Patients with severe sulfa allergies may not be appropriate for use with sulfonylureas.

Patient Education

1. This pill does not make insulin, but it stimulates your pancreas to make more insulin. It is a "cheerleader for the pancreas."
2. Take 30 minutes prior to breakfast and dinner (if ordered BID).
3. Eat consistent food portions at each meal and don't wait more than 5 hours from one meal to the next meal. If it is longer, eat a 15-g carbohydrate snack, such as a piece of fruit.
4. Skipping a meal may cause a low sugar reaction.
5. Carry a fast sugar source with you at all times and especially when exercising, going for a walk, or driving a car.

6. Avoid drinking alcohol, if possible, for the first 3 weeks to assess medication effect on glucose levels.
7. Drink alcohol with food. One beverage for women and two for men per day.
8. Don't double up on the pill if you are going to eat more food. The pill does not work quickly and may cause low blood sugar later in the day.
9. Women planning to get pregnant taking orals often need to go on insulin during pre-conception period. Early planning with OB-GYN and MD is necessary for proper medication and glucose control prior to pregnancy.[6]
10. Carry ID with you that states "I have diabetes" and include MD name and phone number as well as family contact and medications.

Thiazolidinediones

Use

Improve insulin sensitivity by several mechanisms mediated by peroxisome proliferator-activated receptors, gamma that promotes insulin-dependent glucose uptake into adipose tissue and skeletal muscle. TZDs increase levels of adiponectin, which suppresses glucose production by the liver, increases insulin sensitivity by increasing fatty acid oxidation, and decreases the buildup of triglycerides in skeletal muscle, and has an anti-inflammatory effect on the endothelial lining.[7]

Dosage

Check liver enzymes prior to therapy and periodically thereafter. May take 6 to 12 weeks (see **Table 3.1**) for therapy to take effect, so consider increasing dose after this time period.

Possible Side Effects

Edema and weight gain; bone fractures primarily in women at the hand, upper arm, or foot; cold-like symptoms; anemia; or headache.

Possible increased risk of hypoglycemia with use of sulfonylurea or insulin.

Precautions and Considerations[8,9]

Blackbox warning related to heart failure: "TZDs may cause or exacerbate CHF in some patients."

TZDs are contraindicated with patients who have NYHA III or IV heart failure. (NYHA stands for New York Heart Association, which has a classification system for heart failure.) GlaxoSmithKline, the manufacturer of Avandia, states, "Avandia may increase risk of other heart problems if patient taking nitrates or insulin. Use of Avandia with insulin or nitrates is not recommended." TZDs are contraindicated if pregnant or planning to become pregnant and during lactation. Use of TZDs is contraindicated with liver disease and enzymes >2.5 times normal. TZDs may cause ovulation in anovulatory women—discuss family planning.

Patient Education

1. Call MD immediately if sudden weight gain, fluid retention, or shortness of breath.
2. Women who may be anovulatory and premenopausal and who are starting a TZD should discuss family planning.
3. Take the medication regularly, but you may not see a change in the glucose for several weeks.
4. This pill will only help the insulin your body is making work better, so healthy eating and daily activity are very important.
5. Take with or without food.
6. There is increased risk of hypoglycemia with insulin or sulfonylurea use, so carry fast-acting sugar source at all times.
7. Women planning to get pregnant and taking orals often need to go on insulin during the pre-conception period. Early planning with OB-GYN and MD is necessary for proper medication and glucose control prior to pregnancy.
8. Carry ID with you that states "I have diabetes" and include MD name and phone number as well as family contact and medications.

DPP-4 Inhibitors

Use

Allow glucagon-like peptide-1 (GLP-1) and gastric inhibitory polypeptide (GIP) to stimulate pancreas insulin secretion and suppress glucose release by the liver. DPP-4 inhibitors block dipeptidyl peptidase 4, which causes the degradation of GLP-1 and GIP.[10]

Dosage[11,12]

Sitagliptin 100 mg daily. See **Table 3.3**.
Saxagliptin 5 mg daily

Possible Side Effects

Upper respiratory infection, nasopharyngitis, headache, increased risk of hypoglycemia if used with sulfonylureas.

Precautions and Contraindications

See the sitagliptin dosing chart in **Table 3.3** for patients with renal issues and known hypersensitivity to the drugpost marking reports of allergic and hypersensitivity reactions such as anaphylaxis, angioedema, and exfoliative skin conditions including Stevens-Johnson syndrome. No studies in pregnancy or for patients under the age of 18.

Saxagliptin should be decreased to 2.5 mg daily if the patient has a urine creatinine clearance less than or equal to 50 mL/min, or end-stage renal disease (ESRD) requiring hemodialysis. Saxagliptin has

Table 3.3 Renal Dosing with Sitagliptin	
DECREASE DOSE TO 50 MG DAILY	DECREASE DOSE TO 25 MG DAILY IF ON DIALYSIS OR:
CrCl ≥30 to 50 mL/min	CrCl <30 mL/min
Serum Cr ♂ >1.7 to ≤3.0 mg/dL	Serum Cr ♂ >3.0 mg/dL
Serum Cr ♀ >1.5 to ≤2.5 mg/dL	Serum Cr ♀ >2.5 mg/dL

not been studied in patients receiving peritoneal dialysis. It is also recommended to decrease the dose of saxagliptin to 2.5 mg if the patient is also taking cytochrome P450 3A4/5 inhibitors (CYP3A4/5 inhibitors) such as ketoconazole, atazanavir, clarithromycin, indinavir, ritonavir, saquinavir, and telithromycin.

The sulfonylurea dose may need to be decreased to prevent hypoglycemia.

Patient Education

1. Once daily dosing.
2. May increase risk of hypoglycemia with use of sulfonylurea, so take precautions.
3. Stop medication and notify MD immediately if you experience any allergic reaction.
4. Women planning to get pregnant who are taking orals often need to go on insulin during the pre-conception period. Early planning with OB-GYN and MD is necessary for proper medication and glucose control prior to pregnancy.
5. Carry ID with you that states "I have diabetes" and include MD name and phone number as well as family contact and medications.

Alpha Glucosidase Inhibitors[13,14]

Use

Slow down the absorption of carbohydrates through the small intestine, resulting in a decrease in the postprandial glucose level.

Dosage

Patients should take 25 mg with the first bite of breakfast, lunch, and dinner. If patient has GI complaints, he or she may start out with one at the largest meal and increase weekly to TID. Increase dose by 25 mg every 4 to 8 weeks. Check the postprandial glucose to evaluate dose effectiveness. Only use >50 mg TID if patient body weight >60 kg because of the risk of increased serum transaminase.

Possible Side Effects
GI complaints, abdominal pain, diarrhea, flatulence.

Precautions and Contraindications
Dose-related elevation of alanine transaminase (ALT) and/or aspartate aminotransferase (AST), more common in females, reversible, and not associated with liver dysfunction. Check ALT/AST every 3 months during the first year of treatment. No studies with patients who have a SrCr >2 mg/dL. Contraindicated with pregnancy and lactation, cirrhosis, inflammatory bowel disease, or malabsorption disorders and diabetic ketoacidosis.

Patient Education
1. Take with the first bite of each meal.
2. Risk of hypoglycemia increases with use of sulfonylurea or insulin.
3. If hypoglycemia occurs, need to treat with glucose such as glucose gel or tablets; absorption of fruit juice will be delayed as a result of drug effect.
4. GI side effects will diminish over several weeks.
5. Women planning to get pregnant who are taking orals often need to go on insulin during the pre-conception period. Early planning with OB-GYN and MD is necessary for proper medication and glucose control prior to pregnancy.
6. Carry ID with you that states "I have diabetes" and include MD name and phone number as well as family contact and medications.

Meglitinides, Secretagogues[15,16]
Use
Stimulate the pancreas to release insulin rapidly but have a shorter duration than do the sulfonylureas; therefore, less risk of postmeal hypoglycemia. May be beneficial for patients with erratic eating schedules.

Dosage

When starting repaglinide (Prandin), for patients previously not treated or with A1c <8%, starting dose is 0.5 mg with each meal. Start with 1 mg or 2 mg each meal for patients with A1c >8% and previously treated with diabetes medications. In patients with severe renal impairment, start at 0.5 mg dose (no studies conducted on patients with ESRD). When starting nateglinide (Starlix), dose is 120 mg with each meal. Use nateglinide in 60-mg doses if A1c is near goal.

Possible Side Effects

Generally well tolerated with a lower risk of hypoglycemia than with the sulfonylureas.

Precautions and Contraindications

Caution with patients who have impaired liver function and renal function. Consider lower doses and increase doses carefully. Prandin is contraindicated in use with NPH insulin. It is also contraindicated with pregnancy and lactation.

Patient Education

1. Take 1 minute to 30 minutes before a meal.
2. Do not take a pill if you skip the meal.
3. Carry a fast sugar source with you at all times in the event of hypoglycemia.
4. Women planning to get pregnant who are taking orals often need to go on insulin during the pre-conception period. Early planning with OB-GYN and MD is necessary for proper medication and glucose control prior to pregnancy.
5. Carry ID with you that states "I have diabetes" and include MD name and phone number as well as family contact and medications.

Noninsulin Injectable Medications

Incretin Mimetics

Incretins such as GLP-1 and glucose-dependent insulinotropic peptide, also known as GIP, are naturally occurring hormones secreted from the intestine in response to food intake. In the pancreas, incretin hormones act to increase glucose-dependent insulin secretion from beta cells. This action helps to ensure an appropriate insulin response following ingestion of a meal.[17]

Exenatide (BYETTA)[18]

A synthetic version of a protein, exendin-4, was first identified in Gila monster saliva (*Heloderma suspectum*).[19] This lizard hormone is about 50% identical to the GLP-1 hormone in humans.

Use

To be used with patients who have type 2 diabetes only.

Exenatide stimulates the beta cells to release insulin, decreases glucagon release therefore decreasing hepatic glucose release, and slows down gastric emptying, which lowers postprandial levels and increases satiety. Approved for use with metformin, sulfonylureas, or a thiazolidinedione.

Dosage

Start at 5 mcg administered before the morning and evening meals or before the two largest meals of the day (need to be 6 hours apart). Should be administered within 60 minutes of the meal. Do not administer after a meal. After 1 month, increase dose to 10 mcg twice daily based on clinical response. Administer into thigh, abdomen, or upper arm.

Possible Side Effects

GI—nausea, vomiting, diarrhea, dyspepsia (to diminish these side effects patients should inject closer to actual time of eating). Feeling jittery, dizziness, and headache may occur.

Precautions and Contraindications

Contraindicated with type 1 diabetes, ESRD or renal impairment (Cr clearance <30 mL/min), severe GI disease or dysfunction, pregnancy, or lactation. Since 2007, after discussions with the Food and Drug Administration, "observe patients for signs and symptoms of acute pancreatitis" has been added to the package insert. Stop BYETTA immediately if pancreatitis is suspected. May cause hypoglycemia with concomitant use with sulfonylureas. It is recommended to initially decrease sulfonylurea dose by 50% with initiation of BYETTA and adjust dose as necessary.

Patients taking medications requiring rapid absorption should take these medications 1 hour apart from injecting BYETTA because of the gastric slowing effect of BYETTA.

Patient Education

1. Inject into the abdomen, thigh, or upper arm anytime within 60 minutes of morning and evening meals, or before the two main meals of a day, which must be 6 hours apart.
2. Do not administer BYETTA after the meal.
3. Know what to do if you get hypoglycemia (hypoglycemia instructions) especially if you are also taking a sulfonylurea; carry a fast sugar source at all times.
4. If GI symptoms occur, take BYETTA immediately prior to the meal.
5. Call MD for any persistent abdominal pain or vomiting (may be signs and symptoms of pancreatitis).
6. Take oral contraceptives or antibiotics at least 1 hour apart from BYETTA injection.
7. The BYETTA pen is good for 30 days at room temperature once opened.
8. Do not keep the pen needle on the BYETTA pen after use.
9. Store new unused BYETTA pens in the refrigerator.
10. Notify MD if planning to conceive. BYETTA will need to be discontinued (d/c). Early planning with OB-GYN and

MD is necessary for proper medication and glucose control prior to pregnancy.

11. Carry ID with you that states "I have diabetes" and include MD name and phone number as well as family contact and medications.

Amylin

Amylin is a neuroendocrine hormone that is colocated and cosecreted with insulin in the islets of Langerhans.[20]

Pramlintide[21]

Pramlintide (SYMLIN) is an injectable synthetic analog of human amylin.

Use

To be used with patients who have type 1 diabetes or type 2 diabetes requiring insulin. Slows down gastric emptying and decreases glucagon release, both of which result in a lower postprandial glucose level. Also promotes satiety, which may lead to weight loss.

Dosage

Type 1 Adults

Initial dose is 15 mcg subcutaneously into thigh or abdomen immediately prior to a major meal that contains ≥250 k/cal or ≥30 g of carbohydrate. Adjust every 3 to 7 days, if no severe nausea, to a maintenance dose of 45 mcg or 60 mcg. Reduce mealtime insulin by 50% initially to prevent hypoglycemia.

Type 2 Adults

Initial dose is 60 mcg subcutaneously into thigh or abdomen immediately prior to a major meal that contains ≥250 k/cal or ≥30 g of carbohydrate. Adjust every 3 to 7 days, if no severe nausea, to a maintenance dose of 120 mcg. Reduce mealtime insulin by 50% initially to prevent hypoglycemia.

Possible Side Effects

Hypoglycemia, GI complaints, especially nausea, and injection site redness, swelling, or itching.

Precautions and Contraindications

Contraindicated with gastroparesis, hypoglycemia unawareness, pregnancy or lactation, patients who are unwilling to monitor glucose pre and post meal, use with drugs that slow gastric motility, or A1c >9%. Severe hypoglycemia associated with SYMLIN may occur within the first 3 hours following the injection. No studies have been done in patients on dialysis or with hepatic impairment. Do not mix insulin and SYMLIN together.

Patients taking medications requiring rapid absorption should take these medications 1 hour prior or 2 hours after injecting SYMLIN because of the gastric slowing effect of SYMLIN.

Patient Education
1. Inject subcutaneously and do not mix with insulin.
2. Reduce mealtime insulin by 50%.
3. Only inject if the meal contains ≥250 k/cal or ≥30 g of carbohydrate.
4. Inject SYMLIN and insulin at least 2 inches apart.
5. Do not take SYMLIN if you skip a meal or your glucose is too low.
6. Do not use SYMLIN if the liquid is cloudy. Return the vial to the pharmacy.
7. Check your glucose before and 2 hours after each meal and at bedtime.
8. Call for insulin adjustments.
9. Pen or vials can be refrigerated or kept at room temperature for 30 days once opened.
10. Keep unopened vials or pens in the refrigerator.
11. Notify MD if planning to conceive. SYMLIN will need to be d/c. Early planning with OB-GYN and MD is necessary for proper medication and glucose control prior to pregnancy.
12. Carry ID with you that states "I have diabetes" and include MD name and phone number as well as family contact and medications.

Insulin

Considerations prior to initiating insulin:

- Attitude:
  - How does the patient feel about starting insulin? What are his or her concerns or fears?
  - Addressing the patient's cultural beliefs and preconceived ideas about insulin can increase the likelihood that he or she will follow through with your recommendations.
  - Does the patient understand the purpose and need for insulin?
  - Your attitude and the way you approach starting insulin may influence the patient's willingness to start insulin therapy.

- Ability:
  - Visual acuity
  - Dexterity
  - Ability to read, comprehend, literacy
  - Memory

- Possible education needs:
  - Glucose meter
  - Basic diabetes care guidelines
  - Hypoglycemia

- Support:
  - Does the patient have a support person?

- Finances:
  - Which insulin options can the patient afford?

There are two main types of insulin:

- Basal insulin (background insulin)
  - Serves to inhibit glycogenolysis and gluconeogenesis.
  - It has no effect on food.
  - It is released in a slow, steady manner.
- Bolus insulin (nutrition or correction insulin)
  - Given at mealtimes to process carbohydrates
  - Used as a correction insulin to bring the blood glucose back to goal.

Table 3.4   Basal Insulin Options

Types of Basal Insulin	NPH* Novolin Humulin	Glargine† Lantus	Detemir* Levemir
Onset	1–2 hr	2–4 hr	1.6 hr
Peak	4–12	Minimal	Minimal
Duration	Up to 24 hr	Up to 24 hr	Up to 24 hr
Caution	Potential for hypoglycemia at peak	Do not mix with any other insulin	Do not mix with any other insulin
Cost‡	$54–$58	$104	$104

*From: Novo Nordisk. *Novo Nordisk Insulin and Delivery System Portfolio* [brochure]. Bagsværd, Denmark: Novo Nordisk; 2007.
† From: Sanofi-Aventis. *Dosing and Titration Options for Basal and Prandial Insulin* [brochure]. Bridgewater, NJ: Sanofi-Aventis; 2008.
‡ From: Drugstore.com; May 2009. Prices will vary at individual locations and pharmacies.

Basal Insulin

Basal insulin provides about 50%[22] of daily insulin requirements and is relatively continuous over 24 hours. Helps control hepatic glucose output between meals and overnight. All of these types of insulin, listed in **Table 3.4**, can be given once or twice daily.

Basal Insulin Therapy

Starting Basal Insulin for Type 2 Diabetes[23]

1. A1c is not at goal.
2. Fasting glucose levels are elevated.
3. Patient is willing to take one injection.
4. Patient is willing to check fasting glucose.
5. Patient is on maximum oral agents.

Considerations with Starting Basal Insulin

1. Typical starting basal dose is 0.1 (lower body mass index [BMI] or A1c level) to 0.2 unit (higher BMI or A1c level >9) per kilogram of weight.

2. Continue with current oral antidiabetic agents[24] at same doses, except Avandia, which is contraindicated with insulin.[25]
3. Usually given at bedtime, which decreases the fasting glucose and allows daytime oral antidiabetic agents to work.
4. NPH has a peak, which means the patient has a higher risk of hypoglycemia and appropriate patient teaching and cautious adjustments should be implemented.
5. It is recommended when starting basal insulin or increasing the dose that the patient check a glucose reading in the middle of the night to assess for risk of hypoglycemia.

Here is an example of calculating a starting dose of basal insulin: Weight 202 lbs and A1c 9.6:

$$202 \text{ lbs} \div 2.2 \text{ kg} = 92 \text{ kg} \times 0.2 \text{ unit of insulin}$$
$$= 18 \text{ units of basal insulin}$$

Advancing Basal Insulin at Home

There are two options:

1. Patient calls the office weekly for adjustments by MD, nurse practitioner, or physician's assistant.
2. If the patient is capable, he or she may adjust his or her own insulin dose every 3 days until the fasting goal is reached. Typically, this is an adjustment of 1 or 2 units every 3 days until the fasting glucose level is at goal. Individualize your patient's fasting goal; for someone who is labile or elderly, a fasting goal of 120–130 mg/dL may be safer than a goal of 100 mg/dL.

Patient Education for Starting Basal Insulin

1. Take insulin at the same time each day.
2. Do not mix any other insulin with glargine or detemir.
3. Basal insulin has no effect on food, so continue to eat healthfully and be active.
4. Carry a fast sugar source with you at all times.
5. Continue to take your diabetes pills as prescribed.
6. Glargine must be discarded in 28 days after opening.[26] Detemir must be discarded after 6 weeks, and NPH in 30 days.[27]

7. Rotate the injection sites.
8. Carry ID with you that states "I have diabetes" and include MD name and phone number as well as family contact and medications.
9. Call MD as fasting glucose gets close to goal as your diabetes pills may need to be decreased or stopped.

Type 2 Diabetes and Adding Bolus Insulin[28]

1. Fasting glucose is in range.
2. Daytime glucose levels are elevated.
3. A1c is not at goal.
4. Patient basal insulin dose >0.5–0.7 u/kg/day.

Considerations for Adding Bolus Insulin

1. There are several methods to initiate bolus insulin:
   a. Add bolus insulin only to the largest meal of the day by giving 10% of the total daily dose (TDD) as rapid-acting analog and reducing the basal dose by 10%.[29] Example: Patient is currently taking 50 units TDD. Ten percent of 50 units = 5 units. Patient will begin 5 units rapid-acting analog at largest meal and decrease basal by 10% = 45 units basal insulin.
   b. Add bolus insulin to all three meals of the day by taking 0.1 unit/kg and distributing at the meals.[30] Example: 90 kg × 0.1 = 9 units ÷ 3 meals = 3 units at each meal.
2. Discontinue sulfonylureas, exenatide (BYETTA), DPP-4 inhibitors[24] especially when advancing to multiple daily mealtime bolus injections.
3. *Caution:* When using NPH insulin as a basal insulin BID, bolus insulin is given at breakfast and dinner only because of the peak of the morning NPH during lunch time.
4. Carbohydrate counting provides mealtime flexibility for the patient who is capable of carrying out this higher level of management. (See Chapter 4, Medical Nutrition Therapy (MNT) and Exercise.)

   See **Table 3.5** for information on bolus insulin options.

Table 3.5   Bolus Insulins

REGULAR NOVOLIN HUMULIN*	GLULISINE APIDRA†	LISPRO HUMALOG*	ASPART NOVOLOG‡
"Short acting"	"Rapid acting"	"Rapid acting"	"Rapid acting"
Onset: 30 min	Onset: 5–15 min	Onset: 5–15 min	Onset: 10–20 min
Peak: 2–4 hr	Peak: 30–90 min	Peak: 30–90 min	Peak: 40–50 min
Duration: 5–8 hr	Duration: <5 hr	Duration: <5 hr	Duration: 3–5 hr
Cost* $58 Based on vials	Cost $102	Cost $103	Cost $112

*From: Eli Lilly and Company. *Lilly Insulin Time Action Profile* [brochure]. Indianapolis, IN: Eli Lilly and Company; 2008.
† From: Sanofi-Aventis. *Dosing and Titration Options for Basal and Prandial Insulin* [brochure]. Bridgewater, NJ: Sanofi-Aventis; 2008.
‡ From: Novo Nordisk. *Novo Nordisk Insulin and Delivery System Portfolio* [brochure]. Bagsværd, Denmark: Novo Nordisk; 2007.
§ From: Drugstore.com; May 2009. Prices will vary at individual locations and pharmacies.

Patient Education

1. Take lispro[31] or glulisine[32] 15 minutes prior to the meal and aspart[23] 10 minutes prior to the meal. Regular[33] insulin should be taken 30 minutes prior to the meal.
2. Aspart, lispro, and glulisine should be discarded 28 days after opening the vial. Regular insulin should be discarded after opening in 30 days.
3. Rotate the injection sites.
4. Carry a fast sugar source with you at all times.
5. Carry ID with you that states "I have diabetes" and include MD name and phone number as well as family contact and medications.

Mixed-Dose Insulin

Mixed-dose insulin can be used for patients who are unwilling to take more than two injections a day or who require a simpler

Table 3.6   Premixed Insulin Options

	Humulin or Novolin 70/30	Humalog Mix 75/25	NovoLog Mix 70/30	Humalog Mix 50/50
Mixture	70% NPH plus 30% regular	75% lispro protamine plus 25% lispro	70% aspart protamine plus 30% aspart	50% lispro protamine plus 50% lispro
Timing with meal	30 min ac	15 min ac	15 min ac	15 min ac
Cost*	$58	$111	$110	Pen $200

*From: Drugstore.com; May 2009. Prices will vary at individual locations and pharmacies.

regimen because of dexterity, vision, or learning needs. **Table 3.6** lists mixed-dose options.

Considerations with Mixed-Dose Insulin

- Because the vial or pen contains basal and bolus insulin, if you need to increase the basal, you are going to also increase the bolus as well, so there is less flexibility with dose adjustments.
- The patient should try to eat at the same time each day and eat the same portions at each meal to decrease risk of hypoglycemia.
- Mixed-dose insulin is not recommended with type 1 diabetes, if possible, because of lack of flexibility with adjusting the doses.

Starting Twice-Daily Mixed-Dose Insulin

- Use 0.4–0.8 unit/kg to formulate the TDD. Patient should take half at breakfast and half at dinner.[34]
- Example: 195 lbs ÷ 2.2 = 89 kg × 0.6 unit/kg = 53 units TDD ÷ 2 = 27 units at breakfast and 27 units at evening meal.

Patient Education

1. Take Novolin or Humulin 70/30 insulin 30 minutes before breakfast and the evening meal if ordered twice a day.
2. NovoLog Mix 70/30, Humalog Mix 75/25, and Humalog Mix 50/50 should be injected 15 minutes before breakfast and the evening meal if ordered twice a day.
3. NovoLog Mix 70/30, Humalog Mix 75/25, Humalog Mix 50/50, and Humulin or Novolin 70/30 vials should be discarded in 28 days.
4. Rotate the injection sites.
5. Carry a fast sugar source with you at all times.
6. Carry ID with you that states "I have diabetes" and include MD name and phone number as well as family contact and medications.

Type 1 Diabetes

People with type 1 diabetes require daily basal and bolus insulin or they will go into diabetic ketoacidosis. To determine the TDD calculate 0.4 to 0.8 unit/kg/day. Half of the TDD is used as basal insulin and the other half of the TDD is used as bolus mealtime insulin.[35]

Considerations: New Diagnosis

Up to 10% insulin production may still be present in the beta cells, and this is known as the "honeymoon phase." It is recommended to start basal bolus insulin doses conservatively, monitor glucose levels, and adjust doses accordingly because risk of hypoglycemia increases if the patient is in the honeymoon phase. The honeymoon phase may last a few weeks to months and is more common in patients who are in early adulthood vs. in younger children.[36]

Insulin Regimens

Consider the option of NPH and regular insulin for uninsured or underinsured patients. This insulin regimen is not usually recommended for type 1 diabetes because of the increased risk of hypoglycemia.

1. NPH and regular doses need to be split and to be given two thirds in the morning and one third in the evening (patients should take NPH at bedtime preferably to decrease the risk of nocturnal hypoglycemia).
2. Regular insulin is given at breakfast and dinner.
3. There is a higher risk of hypoglycemia with this regimen, and patient education regarding hypoglycemia, mealtimes, and activity is very important.

Example: Patient weight 168 lbs ÷ 2.2 = 76 kg × 0.5 unit insulin = 38 units total daily dose; 25 units should be given in the morning and 13 units in the evening. NPH in the morning = 17 units plus 8 units of regular. For evening meal, NPH 9 units plus 4 units of regular insulin, or if the patient is willing to take three injections a day, move the evening NPH to bedtime to decrease the risk of nocturnal hypoglycemia.

Detemir or Glargine and Rapid-Acting Insulin

This regimen allows for mealtime flexibility, has a lower risk of hypoglycemia, and physiologically mimics the body's usual insulin process better.

1. Calculate the TDD: Weight in kg × 0.4 to 0.8 unit of insulin a day. Divide half for use as basal insulin and the other half into three meals. Example: The patient weighs 154 lbs ÷ 2.2 = 70 kg × 0.5 unit of insulin = 35 units total daily dose ÷ 2 = 17 units basal insulin and 17 ÷ 3 meals = 6 units bolus insulin per meal.
2. Rapid-acting insulin is administered at meals.
3. If the predinner glucose levels are consistently elevated and not related to food or some other factor, the basal insulin may not be effective for 24 hours. The basal insulin dose should be split to BID, morning and evening.[37]
4. If it is appropriate for the patient, teach carbohydrate and correction regimen to provide even more precise insulin dosing.

Mixed-Dose Insulin

Consider the mixed-dose insulin option for those unable or unwilling to take more than two injections a day. This may also be an option for the uninsured person with very limited funds (Humulin or Novolin 70/30).

1. Should be given at breakfast and evening meal.
2. Less flexibility in adjusting basal or bolus insulin doses due to mixture.
3. Less flexibility in mealtimes. Patient should eat at regular times and use consistent portions.

Insulin Pump Therapy

Refer to the section regarding insulin pump therapy in Chapter 7.

1. Only rapid-acting insulin is used in the insulin pump.
2. Basal doses and time frames are programmed into the insulin pump and run continuously.
3. Patient boluses at mealtimes, accounting for carbohydrate and correction needs.
4. Insulin is absorbed at a constant pace, which decreases insulin variability.
5. Allows for the most flexibility with day-to-day life.
6. Consider an endocrinology consult.

Carbohydrate Counting and Correction Scale

See Chapter 4 for information on carbohydrate counting and using the correction scale.

Medication Resources for the Patient

State Pharmacy Assistance Programs: Several states have State Pharmacy Assistance Programs (SPAPs) that help certain people pay for prescription drugs. Each SPAP makes its own rules about how to provide drug coverage to its members. Depending on the patient's state, the SPAP will have different ways of helping him or her pay prescription drug costs. To find out about the SPAPs in a particular state, call 1-800-MEDICARE. Or call your state's State Health Insurance Assistance Program or see the booklet *Medicare Coverage of Diabetes Supplies and Services* at www.medicare.gov/ Publications/Pubs/pdf/11022.pdf.

National programs:

○ Rx Assist Patient Assistance Program Center: www.rxassist.org
○ Together Rx Access: www.togetherrxaccess.com/Tx/jsp/ home.jsp

Diabetes Resource Toolkit

Patient Education

3–1 Injectable Medications (Noninsulin)

3–2 Action Sites of Diabetes Pills

3–3 Diabetes Medicines

3–4 Types of Insulin

3–5 Preparation of Insulin for Injection: Single Dose

3–6 Preparation of Insulin for Injection: Mixed Dose

3–7 Site Selection for Insulin Injection

3–8 How to Give an Insulin Injection

3–9 Hyperglycemia (High Blood Glucose)

3–10 Hypoglycemia (Low Blood Glucose)

Clinical Resources

3–11 Correction Bolus Insulin Needed to Lower Your Blood Glucose

3–12 Meal Bolus Insulin Needed to Cover a Meal

3–13 Adjusting Insulin (Basic Principles)

3–1 Injectable Medications (Noninsulin)

BYETTA (Exenatide)

BYETTA is the first in a new class of medications called incretins, only available by injection and usually used in people with type 2 diabetes to keep blood glucose under control. It is taken twice daily, any time within 60 minutes of eating breakfast and dinner, or it can be given at the two largest meals of the day, but they need to be 6 hours apart. BYETTA is *not* insulin. BYETTA lowers blood glucose in the following ways:

- Stimulates the pancreas to make more insulin
- Lowers the amount of glucose released from your liver
- Helps slow digestion of food, which lowers blood glucose after meals
- May reduce your appetite and help with weight loss

Precautions: May cause nausea or vomiting initially

May cause hypoglycemia (low blood sugar) when used with other diabetes medications

Not recommended for use in people with kidney problems

SYMLIN (Pramlintide)

SYMLIN is a human hormone found to be low in people who don't produce enough natural insulin. It is taken by injection and used in people with type 1 or type 2 diabetes (who require insulin). It is injected with mealtime insulin to lower blood glucose in the following ways:

- Reduces postmeal blood sugar spikes
- Slows digestion, which improves postmeal blood sugars
- May promote weight loss

Scripps Whittier
Diabetes Institute

Precautions: May cause nausea initially

May cause hypoglycemia (low blood sugar) and mealtime insulin dose may need to be reduced by up to 50%—talk with your doctor for dose recommendations

Only use if meal contains at least 30 g of carbohydrate or 250 calories

Do not use if your premeal glucose is low

Scripps Whittier
Diabetes Institute

3–2 ACTION SITES OF DIABETES PILLS

Diabetes medicines are pills that lower blood glucose. These pills are **not** insulin.

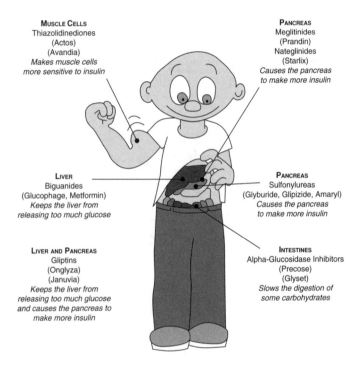

MUSCLE CELLS
Thiazolidinediones
(Actos)
(Avandia)
*Makes muscle cells
more sensitive to insulin*

PANCREAS
Meglitinides
(Prandin)
Nateglinides
(Starlix)
*Causes the pancreas
to make more insulin*

LIVER
Biguanides
(Glucophage, Metformin)
*Keeps the liver from
releasing too much glucose*

PANCREAS
Sulfonylureas
(Glyburide, Glipizide, Amaryl)
*Causes the pancreas
to make more insulin*

LIVER AND PANCREAS
Gliptins
(Onglyza)
(Januvia)
*Keeps the liver from
releasing too much glucose
and causes the pancreas to
make more insulin*

INTESTINES
Alpha-Glucosidase Inhibitors
(Precose)
(Glyset)
*Slows the digestion of
some carbohydrates*

3–3 Diabetes Medicines

It is important for you to know the name and dosage of the medication you are taking. You should not increase, skip, or change your dosage unless you are told to do so by your physician. Women who are taking diabetes pills and are planning to become pregnant should contact their physician.

Generic Name	Brand Name	Dosages Available	Best Time
Tolazamide	Tolinase	100, 200, & 500 mg	Before meals
Tolbutamide	Orinase	500 mg	Before meals
Chlorpropamide	Diabinese	250 mg	Before meals
Glyburide	Diabeta	1.25, 2.5, & 5 mg	Either on an empty stomach or with food
	Micronase	2.5 & 5 mg	
	Glynase PresTab	1.5, 3, & 6 mg	
Glipizide	Glucotrol	5 & 10 mg	Take ½ hour before meal
	Glucotrol XL	2.5, 5, & 10 mg	
Glimepiride	Amaryl	1, 2, & 4 mg	With meals or before breakfast
Repaglinide	Prandin	0.5, 1, & 2 mg	Take ½ hour before meal
Nateglinide	Starlix	60 & 120 mg	Take immediately before meals
Metformin (Hydrochloride)	Glucophage	500, 850, & 1,000 mg	With meals
	Glucophage XR	500 mg	
Acarbose	Precose	25, 50, & 100 mg	With first bite of food

Scripps Whittier Diabetes Institute

(continued)

Generic Name	Brand Name	Dosages Available	Best Time
Miglitol	Glyset	25, 50, & 100 mg	With first bite of food
Rosiglitazone	Avandia	2, 4, & 8 mg	With or without food
Pioglitazone	Actos	15, 30, & 45 mg	With or without food
Sitagliptin	Januvia	25, 50, & 100 mg	With or without food
Saxagliptin	Onglyza	5 mg or 2.5 mg	With or without food

Actoplus = Metformin + Pioglitazone

Avandamet = Metformin + Rosiglitazone

Avandaryl = Rosiglitazone + Glimepiride

Duetact = Pioglitazone + Glimepiride

GlucoVance = Metformin + Glyburide

Janumet = Metformin + Januvia

Metaglip = Metformin + Pioglitazone

PrandiMet = Prandin + Metformin

3–4 TYPES OF INSULIN

	NAME OF INSULIN	STARTS WORKING (ONSET)	WORKS BEST (PEAK)	ENDS (DURATION)
BOLUS	Rapid-acting Apidra (glulisine)* Humalog (lispro)* Novolog (aspart)*	5–15 min	½–1½ hr	3–4 hr
	Short-acting (regular**)	30–60 min	2–4 hr	6–8 hr
BASAL	Intermediate-acting NPH	2–4 hr	6–10 hr	10–18 hr
	Long-acting Lantus (glargine)† Levemir (detemir)†	1–2 hr 1–2 hr	— 	24 hr ± 4 hr Up to 24 hr
COMBINATION	50% N/50% R 50%/50% Humalog 70% N/30% R 75%/25% Humalog Mix 70%/30 % Novolog Mix	Combination of Different Insulins Action Varies***		

*Should be given 0–15 minutes before meal.

**Should be given 30 minutes before meal.

***Discuss specific action times with your healthcare provider.

†Cannot be mixed in syringe with other insulin(s).

Scripps Whittier
Diabetes Institute

3–5 PREPARATION OF INSULIN FOR INJECTION: SINGLE DOSE

1. Wash hands with warm, soapy water.

2. If using cloudy insulin (NPH, 70/30, 75/25, or 50/50), roll bottle between hands.

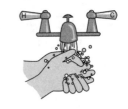

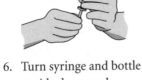

3. Clean rubber stopper of insulin bottle with alcohol.

4. Fill syringe with amount of air equal to the number of units of insulin you will be giving.

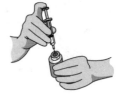

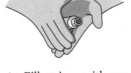

5. Insert the needle into the bottle and push air into the insulin bottle.

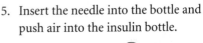

6. Turn syringe and bottle upside down and withdraw your dose of insulin.

3–6 PREPARATION OF INSULIN FOR INJECTION: MIXED DOSE

Follow steps 1, 2, and 3 the same as for single dose.

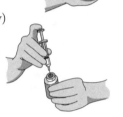

4. Fill syringe with air equal to the number of units of NPH (cloudy) insulin you will give. Insert the needle into NPH bottle. Remove needle from bottle.

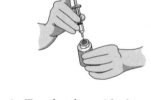

5. Fill syringe with air equal to the number of units of fast-acting (clear) insulin (Apidra, Humalog, Novalog, Regular) you will give. Insert needle into the fast-acting insulin bottle and push air into bottle. Do not remove needle!

6. Turn bottle upside down. Draw out units of fast-acting (clear) insulin. Remove needle from fast-acting bottle.

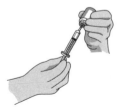

7. Insert needle into NPH (cloudy) insulin. Draw out units of NPH insulin, until you have a total of units of insulin in the syringe. Remove needle from bottle.

Note: Lantus and Levemir cannot be mixed with any other insulin.

Scripps Whittier
Diabetes Institute

©2009

3–7 SITE SELECTION FOR INSULIN INJECTION

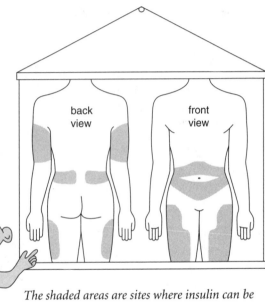

back
view

front
view

The shaded areas are sites where insulin can be given.

- The stomach is the best site for insulin absorption.
- Avoid injecting insulin next to the belly button.

3–8 HOW TO GIVE AN INSULIN INJECTION

1. Clean the skin where the shot is to be given. The best place to give the injection is in your abdomen.

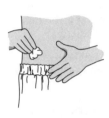

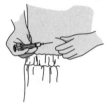

2. Pinch up a large area of skin. Pick up the syringe with the other hand and hold it as you would a pencil. Put the needle straight into the skin (90º angle). Be sure to insert the needle all the way.

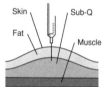

3. Inject the insulin by pushing the plunger all the way down, using less than 5 seconds to give the dose. Wait 10 seconds before removing the needle.

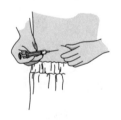

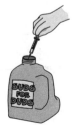

4. Use the syringe only once. **Ask your doctor how you should dispose of your syringe as many states have new regulations regarding syringe disposal.

Scripps Whittier
Diabetes Institute

3–9 Hyperglycemia (High Blood Glucose)

Causes: Too much carbohydrate, not enough medication, illness, or stress

Onset: Gradual, may progress to diabetic coma

Blood Sugar: Above 180 mg/dL

Symptoms

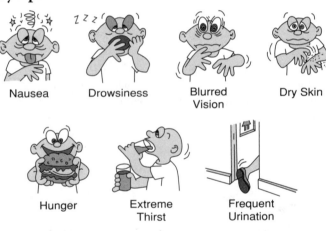

Nausea

Drowsiness

Blurred Vision

Dry Skin

Hunger

Extreme Thirst

Frequent Urination

Recommended Action

Test Blood Sugar

Call Your Diabetes Educator/Doctor

If over 250 mg/dL for several tests

3–10 HYPOGLYCEMIA (LOW BLOOD GLUCOSE)

CAUSES: Too little carbohydrate, too much insulin or diabetes medicine, extra exercise, alcohol

ONSET: Sudden, may progress to insulin shock

BLOOD SUGAR: Below 70 mg/dL

Symptoms

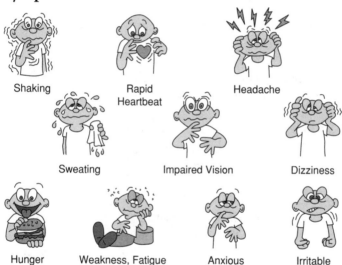

Shaking

Rapid Heartbeat

Headache

Sweating

Impaired Vision

Dizziness

Hunger

Weakness, Fatigue

Anxious

Irritable

Recommended Action

Drink
4 oz. of juice or 8 oz. milk, or eat several hard candies

Test Blood Sugar
If symptoms don't stop, call your doctor

Within 30 Min.
after symptoms end, eat a snack of a peanut butter or meat sandwich and a glass of milk

3–11 CORRECTION BOLUS INSULIN NEEDED TO LOWER YOUR BLOOD GLUCOSE

This is the amount of *Apidra, Humalog, Novolog,* or Regular insulin needed to bring the blood glucose to a desired target.

The 1700 Rule

1. Add up <u>all the insulin</u> in a day (short and long acting). This is called your Total Daily Dose (TDD).
2. Divide 1700 by the TDD.
3. The result is how much 1 unit of *Apidra, Humalog, or Novolog* will lower your blood glucose.

1700 Rule: $\dfrac{1700}{\text{TDD (24 hours)}}$ = the amount 1 unit of *Apidra, Humalog, or Novolog* will lower your blood glucose.

Sample:

Levemir = 20 units daily
+ Humalog = 16 units daily
TDD = 36 units

$\dfrac{1700}{36} = 47$

1 unit *Apidra, Humalog, or Novolog* will lower the blood glucose 47 points.

Note: If on regular insulin, use 1500 instead of 1700.

3–12 Meal Bolus Insulin Needed to Cover a Meal

This is the amount of *Apidra, Humalog, Novolog,* or Regular insulin needed to cover the carbohydrates in a meal. This is where accurate carbohydrate counting comes into play.

The 500 Rule

1. Add up <u>all the insulin in a day</u> (short and long acting). This is called the Total Daily Dose (TDD).
2. Divide 500 by the TDD.
3. The result is the amount of total carbohydrate covered by 1 unit of *Apidra, Humalog, or Novolog.*

500 Rule: $\dfrac{500}{\text{Total Insulin (24 hours)}}$ = Grams carbohydrate covered by one unit of *Apidra, Humalog, or Novolog*

Sample: Lantus = 20 units daily

$\dfrac{\text{+ Humalog = 16 units daily}}{\text{TDD = 36 units}}$

$\dfrac{500}{36} = 14$

1 unit *Apidra, Humalog, or Novolog* covers 14 grams of carbohydrate. (For convenience you may round-off to 15 grams of carbohydrate.)

Note: If on regular insulin, use 450 instead of 500.

3–13 Adjusting Insulin (Basic Principles)

Which Insulin Should I Adjust?

The following table shows how to adjust the type of insulin.

Out of Range Blood Glucose (Not explained by food, illness, exercise, or stress.)	Value	Pattern of Adjustment* (Start by adding 1–2 units. Watch your blood glucose for 2–3 days before making another change. It is better to change 1 dose at a time.)
If your fasting blood glucose is:	High	⇧ PM or bedtime basal
	Low	⇩ PM or bedtime basal
Before lunch:	High	⇧ morning bolus insulin
	Low	⇩ morning bolus insulin
Before dinner:	High	⇧ lunchtime bolus insulin
	Low	⇩ lunchtime bolus insulin
After meals (1½ to 2 hr):	High	⇧ Check accuracy of carbohydrate counting (ratio, portion size, and actual carbohydrate amount)
	Low	⇩ Decrease bolus insulin
Before bedtime:	High	⇧ dinner bolus insulin
	Low	⇩ dinner bolus insulin
During the night:	Low	⇩ Need further testing to determine the cause

☞ Scripps Whittier
Diabetes Institute

References

1. American Diabetes Association. Standards of medical care in diabetes—2009. *Diabetes Care.* 2009;32:s13–s61.

2. Hirsch I, Bergenstal RM, Parkin CG, Wright E, Buse JB. A real world approach to insulin therapy in primary care practice. *Clin Diabetes.* 2005;23:78–86.

3. Rx List. Glucophage, glucophage XR. Available at: http://www.rxlist .com/glucophage-drug.htm. Accessed October 26, 2009.

4. Diabetes Mall. Medications: sulfonylureas. Available at: http://diabetesnet .com/diabetes_treatments/sulfonylureas.php. Accessed October 26, 2009.

5. Rx List. Glucotrol. Available at: http://www.rxlist.com/glucotrol-drug. htm. Accessed October 26, 2009.

6. Barss V, Repke J. Patient information: care during pregnancy for women with type 1 or 2 diabetes. Available at: http://www.uptodate .com/patients/content/topic.do?topicKey=~X1_z7ZpZvSOGF& selectedTitle=2~148&source=search_result. Accessed October 26, 2009.

7. Wilding J. Thiazolidinediones, insulin resistance and obesity: finding a balance. *Int J Clin Pract.* October 2006;60(10):1272–1280.

8. GlaxoSmithKline. Avandia: prescribing information. Available at: http:// us.gsk.com/products/assets/us_avandia.pdf. Accessed October 26, 2009.

9. Takeda Pharmaceuticals North America. Actos: prescribing information. Available at: http://www.actos.com/actos/home.aspx. Accessed October 26, 2009.

10. PharmiWeb Solutions. DPP-4 inhibitors Galvus and Januvia will be the first oral drugs tackling type 2 diabetes via the incretin response: how do they compare? Available at: http://www.pharmiweb.com/ features/feature.asp?ROW_ID=908. Accessed October 26, 2009.

11. Merck and Co. Januvia: prescribing information. Available at: http:// www.januvia.com/sitagliptin/januvia/consumer/prescribing- information-for-januvia/index.jsp?WT.svl=1. Accessed October 26, 2009.

12. Bristal-Myers Squibb and AstraZeneca Pharmaceuticals: prescribing information. Available at: http://packageinserts.bms.com/pi/pi_ onglyza.pdf. Accessed December 16, 2009.

13. Pfizer Pharmaceuticals. Glyset: prescribing information. Available at: http://www.pfizer.com/files/products/uspi_glyset.pdf. Accessed October 26, 2009.

14. Bayer HealthCare Pharmaceuticals. Precose: prescribing information. Available at: http://www.univgraph.com/Bayer/inserts/Precose.pdf. Accessed October 26, 2009.

15. Novo Nordisk. Prandin: prescribing information. Available at: http://www.prandin.com/docs/prandin_insert.pdf. Accessed October 26, 2009.

16. Novartis. Starlix: prescribing information. Available at: http://www.pharma.us.novartis.com/product/pi/pdf/Starlix.pdf. Accessed October 26, 2009.

17. Gautier JF, Choukem SP, Girard J. Physiology of incretins (GIP and GLP-1) and abnormalities in type 2 diabetes. *Diabetes Metab.* 2008;34:S65–S72.

18. Byetta: prescribing information. Available at: http://www.byetta.com. Accessed November 10, 2009.

19. Wikipedia. Gila monster. Available at: http://en.wikipedia.org/wiki/Gila_monster. Accessed October 26, 2009.

20. Wikipedia. Amylin. Available at: http://en.wikipedia.org/wiki/Amylin. Accessed October 26, 2009.

21. Amylin Pharmaceuticals. SYMLIN: prescribing information. Available at: http://www.symlin.com/pdf/SYMLIN-pi-combined.pdf. Accessed October 26, 2009.

22. Mooradian AD, et al. Narrative review: a rational approach to starting insulin therapy. *Ann Intern Med.* 2006;145:125–134.

23. Hirsch I, Bergenstal RM, Parkin CG, Wright E, Buse JB. A real world approach to insulin therapy in primary care practice. *Clin Diabetes.* 2005;23:78–86.

24. Mazze R, Strock E, Simonson G, Bergenstal RM. *Staged Diabetes Management Quick Guide: Prevention, Detection and Treatment of Diabetes in Adults.* 4th ed. Minneapolis, MN: Matrex; 2007:3–29.

25. GlaxoSmithKline. Avandia: prescribing information. Available at: http://us.gsk.com/products/assets/us_avandia.pdf. Accessed October 26, 2009.

26. Sanofi-Aventis. Lantus: prescribing information. Available at: http://www.lantus.com. Accessed October 26, 2009.

27. Novo Nordisk. *Novo Nordisk Insulin and Delivery System Portfolio* [brochure]. Bagsværd, Denmark: Novo Nordisk; 2007.

28. Mazze R, Strock E, Simonson G, Bergenstal RM. *Staged Diabetes Management Quick Guide: Prevention, Detection and Treatment of Diabetes in Adults.* 4th ed. Minneapolis, MN: Matrex; 2007:3–29.

29. Hirsch I, Bergenstal RM, Parkin CG, Wright E, Buse JB. A real world approach to insulin therapy in primary care practice. *Clin Diabetes.* 2005;23:78–86.

30. Mazze R, Strock E, Simonson G, Bergenstal RM. *Staged Diabetes Management Quick Guide: Prevention, Detection and Treatment of Diabetes in Adults.* 4th ed. Minneapolis, MN: Matrex; 2007:3–29.

31. Eli Lilly and Company. *Lilly Insulin Time Action Profile* [brochure]. Indianapolis, Ind: Eli Lilly and Company; 2008.

32. Sanofi-Aventis. *Dosing and Titration Options for Basal and Prandial Insulin* [brochure]. Bridgewater, NJ: Sanofi-Aventis; 2008.

33. Novo Nordisk. *Novo Nordisk Insulin and Delivery System Portfolio* [brochure]. Bagsværd, Denmark: Novo Nordisk; 2007.

34. Edelman S, Henry R. *Diagnosis and Management of Type 2 Diabetes.* 8th ed. West Islip, NY: Professional Communications, Inc.; 2008.

35. Bhargava A. Insulin therapy: the question this issue. *Insulin.* July 2008;3(3):189.

36. Beaser R. *Joslin's Diabetes Deskbook: A Guide for Primary Care Providers.* 2nd ed. Lippincott Williams & Wilkins and Joslin Diabetes Center; Philadelphia, PA; 2007:284.

37. Porcellati F, Rossetti P, Busciantella N, et al. Comparison of pharmacokinetics and dynamics of the long acting insulin analogs glargine and detemir at steady states in type 1 diabetes: a double-blind randomized, crossover study. *Diabetes Care.* 2007;30:2447–2452.

4 ■ Medical Nutrition Therapy (MNT) and Exercise

Eating healthy foods and daily activity are truly the foundation for good health whether a person has diabetes or not. There is no such thing as a "diabetic diet." It is a matter of eating healthy foods and watching the food portions. When you talk to your patients about nutrition and diabetes, it is important to share the information with the patient's family members too because they are at risk for developing diabetes as well (type 2 diabetes). Multiple clinical trials have shown glycemic and metabolic improvement with nutritional support from a registered dietitian. MNT, when delivered by a registered dietitian according to nutrition practice guidelines, is reimbursed as part of the Medicare program.

Clinical Effectiveness of Nutrition Therapy[1]

- Glycemic control
  - A1c decreases by 1–2%
  - Fasting blood sugar decreases by 50–100 mg/dL
- Lipids
  - Total cholesterol decreases 10–13% (24–32 mg/dL)
  - Low-density lipoprotein (LDL) decreases 12–16% (15–25 mg/dL)
  - Triglycerides decrease 8% (15–17 mg/dL)
- Hypertension
  - Systolic decreases an average of 5 mm Hg
  - Diastolic decreases an average of 2 mm Hg

General Nutrition Guidelines

Patients should follow these general nutrition guidelines:

- Eat three *balanced* meals per day.
- Space meals no more than 5 hours apart; if longer time, eat a snack.
- Maintain a healthy weight.
- Be physically active on most days.
- Eat consistent amounts of carbohydrate portions at each meal.
- Choose healthy fats.
- Eat lean protein choices.

Calculating Caloric Needs[2]

Patients need 11 kcal/pound of ideal body weight for weight maintenance with the following considerations:

- Moderately active add 20% to this total
- Very active add 40% to this total
- Subtract 500 kcal per day for weight loss
- For pregnant women add 300 kcal per fetus
- For lactating women add 500 kcal

Table 4.1 shows the recommended percentage of daily calories from each of the major food nutrient categories.

Table 4.1   Recommended Percentage of Daily Calories

Carbohydrates	Protein	Fat
45–65% of total daily calories	15–20% of total daily calories	25–30% of total daily calories

Carbohydrates

Carbohydrates should make up 45–65% of total calories. It is not recommended to have <130 g/day.[3]

Sources: 1 serving = 15 g carbohydrate

- Fruits
- Milk, yogurt, ice cream
- Starch: breads, cereal and grains, starchy vegetables, beans, peas, lentils, crackers
- The goal is to eat complex carbohydrates that are higher in fiber and to eat consistent carbohydrate portions at each meal

Table 4.2 shows the amount of carbohydrate per meal with 50% of the calories from carbohydrates.

Should be individualized based on activity and metabolic needs.

Protein

Protein should comprise 15–20% of a meal.[3] There are 7 g of protein per ounce of protein.

Sources:

- Lean meats such as poultry without the skin, fish, lean beef "choice" or "select" grades (round, sirloin, chuck, loin), lean or extra lean ground beef with no more than 15% fat, lean pork (tenderloin, loin chop), low-salt turkey and sandwich meats[4]
- Eggs
- Tofu
- Cheese—try reduced fat or skim
- Cottage cheese—try low fat

Table 4.3 shows an example of the amount of protein per meal with 20% of calories from protein.

Table 4.2 Example Calculating 50% Carbohydrate				
1,200 calorie	1,500 calorie	1,800 calorie	2,000 calorie	2,200 calorie
50 g carbs/ meal	62 g carbs/ meal	75 g carbs/ meal	83 g carbs/ meal	92 g carbs/ meal

Table 4.3	Example Calculating 20% Protein			
1,200 calorie	1,500 calorie	1,800 calorie	2,000 calorie	2,200 calorie
20 g/meal equals 3 ounces of protein	25 g/meal equals 3.5 ounces of protein	30 g/meal equals 4 ounces of protein	33 g/meal equals 4.5 ounces of protein	37 g/meal equals 5 ounces of protein

Fat

Fat should comprise 25–30% of total calories at a meal, and <7% should come from saturated fat.[3]

Healthy sources of fat:

- Monounsaturated
  - Olive oil
  - Peanut oil
  - Canola oil
  - Avocados
  - Nuts, seeds
- Polyunsaturated
  - Vegetable oils (safflower, soy, sunflower, corn, cottonseed)
  - Walnuts
- Omega-3 fatty acids
  - Salmon, mackerel, herring, tuna, rainbow trout
  - Flaxseed, wheat germ
  - Walnuts/pumpkin seeds

Unhealthy sources of fat:

- Saturated: Goal is <1 g/100 calories
  - Animal products—fatty meats like bacon, ribs, sausage
  - Whole milk
  - Lard, butter
  - Coconut or palm oil

Table 4.4	Example Calculating 30% Fat			
1,200 calorie	1,500 calorie	1,800 calorie	2,000 calorie	2,200 calorie
13 g/meal	17 g/meal	20 g/meal	22 g/meal	24 g/meal

- Trans-fat: Goal is zero
  - Partially hydrogenated fats, which are present in many cakes, cookies, donuts, crackers, margarine, and fried foods
- Dietary cholesterol: Goal is <300 mg/day. If LDL is 100 mg, limit cholesterol to <200 mg/day
  - Lard, butter
  - Fatty meats

Table 4.4 shows an example of the amount of fat calories per meal with 30% of calories coming from fat.

Sodium Considerations[5]

- Reduce dietary sodium intake to 2,300 mg/day.
- 1,500 mg/day reduction may be as effective as a single drug used to treat hypertension.
- Average systolic blood pressure (SBP) reduction range 2–8 mm Hg.
- African Americans especially have a good response to lower sodium intake.

Vitamins and Minerals

- Chromium,[6] potassium, magnesium,[7] vitamin D, and possibly zinc deficiency may aggravate carbohydrate intolerance.
- Serum levels can readily detect the need for potassium, vitamin D, or magnesium replacement, but detecting deficiency of zinc and chromium is more difficult.
- Vitamin D has been shown to improve the body's ability to use insulin; a lack of vitamin D in the body has been shown to lead to higher chances of getting type 2 diabetes.[8]

Fiber[9]

AGE	<50 YR	>50 YR
Men	38 g/day	30 g/day
Women	25 g/day	21 g/day

- Benefits
  - Decreases cholesterol
  - Improves postmeal glucose levels by slowing absorption of food
  - Promotes satiety
  - Lowers risk of digestive conditions
- Foods high in fiber
  - Nuts and seeds
  - Whole grains
  - Fruits and vegetables
  - Beans, peas, and legumes

Alcohol

- May cause hypoglycemia especially with patients taking insulin or sulfonylureas because of inhibition of hepatic glucose release
- Should be consumed with food
- Unless contraindicated, can be consumed at the following rates:
  - Men: 2 drinks daily
  - Women: 1 drink daily
- 1 drink equals
  - 12 oz. beer
  - 5 oz. wine
  - 1.5 oz. distilled spirits

Carbohydrate Counting and Mealtime Insulin

There are two methods of carbohydrate counting: basic carbohydrate counting and advanced carbohydrate counting.

Basic Carbohydrate Counting

- Appropriate for someone who is unable to comprehend mathematical figures (literacy or language barriers) or someone who is not willing to do advanced carbohydrate counting.
- Teach which foods contain carbohydrates and appropriate portion size.
- The plate method is easy to comprehend and use by those who are unable to read food labels or measure portions. **Figure 4.1** is an example of the plate method for weight control.

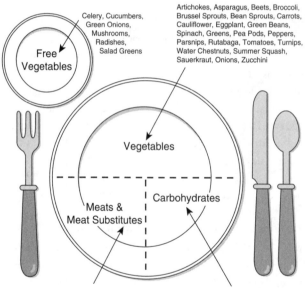

Celery, Cucumbers, Green Onions, Mushrooms, Radishes, Salad Greens

Artichokes, Asparagus, Beets, Broccoli, Brussel Sprouts, Bean Sprouts, Carrots, Cauliflower, Eggplant, Green Beans, Spinach, Greens, Pea Pods, Peppers, Parsnips, Rutabaga, Tomatoes, Turnips, Water Chestnuts, Summer Squash, Sauerkraut, Onions, Zucchini

Free Vegetables

Vegetables

Carbohydrates

Meats & Meat Substitutes

Poultry (Chicken, Turkey), No Skin Fish, Lean Cuts of Beef, Pork, Lamb, Veal (trim fat and Bake, Broil, Boil or BBQ), Low-fat cheese, Eggs, Peanut Butter

Fruit (fresh, canned in juice), Milk, Low-fat Yogurt (Plain or artificially sweetened), Bread, Tortillas, Rolls, English Muffins, Bagels, Crackers, Waffles, Pancakes, Muffin, Hamburger and Hot Dog Buns, Potato, Rice, Pasta, Noodles, Corn, Peas, Sweet Potato, Lima Beans, Dried Peas and Beans, (Pinto, Kidney, Garbanzo), Lentils, Winter Squash

For weight control, fats should be used sparingly (e.g., margarine, oil, mayonnaise, salad dressing, gravy, sour cream, cream cheese, avocado, seeds, nuts).

■ Figure 4.1 The Plate Method
Courtesy of the Scripps Whittier Diabetes Institute.

- Carbohydrate portions should be consistent at each meal.
- Insulin dose should be fixed at each meal. Typical starting dose is 1 unit of rapid-acting or fast-acting insulin for every 15 g of carbohydrate.[10] Example: If the patient eats 60 g of carbohydrate per meal, he or she would take 4 units of rapid-acting or fast-acting insulin at each meal.
- To assess the effectiveness of the insulin dose ask the patient to check a few premeal and 2-hr postmeal glucose levels. The postmeal glucose should be no more than 30–50 mg/dL higher than the premeal glucose value.[11]

Advanced Carbohydrate Counting

- Allows patient to be flexible with mealtimes and foods.
- Teach which foods contain carbohydrate, portion sizes, and food label reading.
- To calculate the amount of carbohydrate covered by 1 unit of mealtime insulin, the total daily dose (TDD) of insulin is divided by 450 (if using regular insulin) or 500 (if using rapid-acting insulin).[10] Example: The patient takes a total of 40 units of insulin a day and uses a rapid-acting insulin at meals, so $500 \div 40 = 13$ g. Therefore, the patient would take 1 unit of rapid-acting insulin for every 13 g of carbohydrates.

Considerations with Advanced Carbohydrate Counting

- Fiber: If the total fiber amount is more than 5 g, subtract half of the amount of fiber from the total carbohydrate.[10]
- Example: Total carbohydrate is 22 g – 4 g of fiber (half of 8 g) = 18 g total carbohydrate to be counted for a serving.

Table 4.5 is a food label that shows sufficient fiber content to be subtracted from the total carbohydrate.

Correction Bolus

- Determines the amount of insulin added to or subtracted from a bolus to correct a glucose that is above or below target. The

Table 4.5   Example Food Label

Food Label	
Serving Size	1 cup
Servings per container	2
Calories	260
Total Fat	8 g
Total Carbohydrate	22 g
Dietary Fiber	8 g
Protein	25 g

premeal glucose goal should be individualized, but in general a goal of 100 mg/dL or 110 mg/dL is acceptable.

- Divide 1,700 (if using rapid-acting insulin) or 1,500 (if using regular insulin) by the TDD of insulin.[10]
- Example: The patient TDD is 40 units of insulin a day and the patient is using rapid-acting insulin, so 1,700 ÷ 40 = 43 mg/dL. Therefore, 1 unit of rapid-acting insulin will drop the glucose 43 mg/dL.

Example Using the Mealtime Bolus and the Correction Scale

1. TDD = 40 units. As determined earlier, the patient will take 1 unit of rapid-acting mealtime insulin for every 13 g of carbohydrate, and 1 unit of rapid-acting insulin will drop the glucose by 43 mg/dL. The patient's premeal goal is 100 mg/dL.
2. Total amount of carbohydrate to be consumed at dinner is 75 g; therefore, 75 g ÷ 13 g = 6 units of rapid-acting insulin for the 75 g of carbohydrate.
3. The premeal glucose is 240 mg/dL, so 240 mg/dL (premeal glucose) − 100 mg/dL (premeal glucose goal) = 140 mg/dL above goal.
4. 140 mg/dL ÷ 43 mg/dL = 3 units of rapid-acting insulin needed to correct the glucose to the goal of 100 mg/dL.

5. Total amount of rapid-acting insulin to be injected by patient prior to meal is as follows:

Mealtime insulin	6 units
Correction insulin	+ 3 units
	9 units total

Nutrition Resources

Institute of Medicine of the National Academies Dietary Reference Intake: http://fnic.nal.usda.gov/nal_display/index.php?info_center=4&tax_level=2&tax_subject=256&topic_id=1342

American Dietetic Association: www.eatright.org

MyPyramid from the United States Department of Agriculture: www.mypyramid.gov

Exercise

Strategies for Self-Directed Exercise Instruction

- What does the patient enjoy doing?
- Is the patient thinking about exercising?
- Identify barriers to exercising.
- Help with realistic and practical goal setting.

Benefits[10]

- Reduces stress.
- Lowers blood pressure.
- May lower LDL and triglycerides and increase high-density lipoprotein (HDL).
- Fights osteoporosis, decreases joint stiffness, increases flexibility, increases balance.
- Induces weight loss, increases muscle mass.
- Is a natural sleep aid.
- Lowers blood glucose, improves insulin sensitivity.
- Is a mild antidepressant, improves self-esteem.
- Improves mental alertness.

- When used three to five times a week, reduces risk of heart attack and stroke.
- Clinical studies show consistent exercise for 8 weeks lowers the A1c 0.66% in patients with type 2 diabetes even if there is no weight loss. The more intense the level of exercise, the greater the A1c drop over the 8 weeks.

Physical Assessment[10]

- Prior to the patient engaging in an exercise program, assess for any microvascular or macrovascular complications.
- Exercise stress test is recommended for:
  - Known or suspected cerebrovascular disease >35 yr of age
  - Age >25 yr and type 2 for 10 yr or type 1 for 15 yr
  - Autonomic neuropathy, peripheral vascular disease, micro-vascular disease

ADA Exercise Recommendations[12]

- At least 150 min/week of moderate-intensity aerobic activity.
- Resistance training three times a week in the absence of contraindications, three sets of 8–10 repetitions. Older adults should maintain resistance training with one set of 8 to 10 exercises for each major muscle group two to three times a week for 8 weeks to allow connective tissues to adapt before increasing sets.
- Avoid more than 2 consecutive days off from exercise.
- Start slowly and work up to recommendations if patient is inactive or elderly.

Precautions[13]

Patients should take the following precautions:

- Check their blood glucose before (it is recommended to check 30 min prior to the activity and 5 min prior to activity to assess glucose trending), during (long bouts), and after exercise.

- Keep a source of rapidly acting carbohydrate available during exercise.
- The abdomen is the best place to inject insulin. Injecting insulin in the arms or legs may cause rapid absorption in the arms or legs, which may cause hypoglycemia during exercise.
- Avoid exercising during peak insulin action.
- Consume adequate fluids before, during, and after exercise (consumption of carbohydrate 30 min after intense exercise restores glycogen levels to lower the risk of hypoglycemia later).
- Practice good foot care and wear properly fitting shoes and socks.
- Carry medical identification.
- Those who have type 1 diabetes and use an insulin pump should:
  - Drop basal rate 50% 1 hr prior to exercising and consider reducing basal at bedtime by 20%.
  - Consider cutting back 50% on meal bolus if exercising around mealtime.[14]
  - These are general guidelines, but each person will need to adjust his or her insulin doses based upon individual glucose responses.

Specific Populations[10]

- Cardiac problems
  - Consider cardiac rehab program.
  - Rhythmic exercises using lower extremities (walking, cycling, rowing, swimming) recommended at moderate intensity.
  - Avoid hypertensive responses (260/125 mm Hg).
  - Avoid lifting, straining anything that would cause Valsalva maneuver.
  - Upper extremity exercises tend to increase SBP.

- Peripheral arterial disease: the patient may experience ischemic pain during physical activity as a result of insufficient oxygen/blood supply.
  - Walking program may improve intermittent claudication, increase muscles' oxidative capacity, increase capillary density, and therefore decrease pain.
  - Walk/rest interval training = greater exercise tolerance.
  - Conversation, music can divert attention from mild pain; when pain accelerates, patients should stop, rest, and start up again.
- Retinopathy—nonproliferative
  - Mild:
    - No restrictions; exercise may improve early stages with positive effects on blood pressure and HDL, reducing macular edema.
  - Moderate:
    - Caution advised, especially with weight-bearing exercises/activities.
  - Severe:
    - Avoid activities that jar the head or increase SBP.
  - Proliferative retinopathy:
    - No Valsalva, head jarring, or any strenuous activity.
- Nephropathy
  - Light weights may help with bone loss.
  - Aerobic activities as tolerated.
- Neuropathy—peripheral
  - Caution with foot injuries.
  - Consider non-weight-bearing activities.
  - Range of motion exercises.
  - Chair and balance exercises will be helpful.
  - Use proper foot wear.
  - Autonomic neuropathy:
    - Caution with hypo/hypertension—monitor blood pressure

- Hypoglycemic unawareness, ask patient to monitor glucose levels more frequently
- Avoid high-impact or heavy lifting activities
- Visual impairment
  - Stationary cycling
  - Swimming with lane markers
  - Treadmill walking
  - Dancing with a partner as a guide

Exercise Resources

Diabetes Exercise and Sports Association: www.diabetes-exercise.org/

Diabetes Training Camp: www.diabetestrainingcamp.com

Biking: www.teamtype1.org

Insulindependence: www.insulindependence.org

Triabetes: www.triabetes.org

Insulin Factor: www.insulinfactor.com

Diabetes Resource Toolkit

Patient Education

4–1 Heart-Healthy Eating Guidelines

4–2 Estimating Portion Sizes

4–3 Weight Loss Tips

4–4 What Are the Sources of Carbohydrates in the Diet?

4–5 Sample Menu 1: 1,500 Calories (1,600 Calories with Snack)

4–6 Sample Menu 2: 1,500 Calories (1,600 Calories with Snack)

4–7 Sample Menu 1: 1,800 Calories (2,000 Calories with Snack)

4–8 Sample Menu 2: 1,800 Calories (2,000 Calories with Snack)

4–9 Make Your Plate Look Like This!

4–10 Make Your Plate Look Like This for Weight Control!

4–1 Heart-Healthy Eating Guidelines

- When following a heart-healthy diet, it is important to reduce daily total fat and saturated fat intake. Ask your dietitian what level is right for you.
- People with coronary heart disease, diabetes, or high LDL cholesterol should decrease saturated and trans fat to no more than 7% of calories. This amounts to no more than 16 grams of saturated trans fat for a 2,000-calorie per day diet. Saturated fats are found in butter, meat, whole milk, cheese, sour cream, bacon, lard, palm and coconut oils. Trans fats are found in margarine, shortening, baked goods, and desserts.
- Limit your average total daily cholesterol intake to less than 200–300 mg. Eggs and shellfish can be a major source of dietary cholesterol, but they are fairly low in saturated fat and total fat. Egg whites have no fat and no cholesterol.
- Heart-healthy fats such as canola oil, olive oil, fatty fish, and nuts are good choices. But beware of their calories and portion appropriately.
- Benecol, Take Control, and Smart Balance Omega Plus are margarine brands that can help lower cholesterol. They contain a plant sterol that binds cholesterol in the intestines so that it is not absorbed.
- Choose brands that contain no trans fatty acids, such as SmartBeat margarine or SmartBeat vegetable shortening.
- Eat fish 2 or 3 times a week, especially those high in omega-3 fatty acids.
- Eat lean meat, fish, and skinless poultry. Purchase lean cuts, trim off visible fat, and discard the fat that cooks out of the meat. The Select grade is the leanest cut of meat.
- Limit organ meats such as liver, brains, chitterlings, kidney, heart, gizzard, and sweet breads.

Barbara Widmer Diabetes Institute

- Use cooking methods that require little or no fat: bake, broil, roast, steam, poach, boil, barbecue, sauté, stir-fry, or microwave. Avoid frying foods. Vegetable spray coatings, nonstick pans, crock pots, or clay pots are some tools you can use.
- Minimize adding fats like butter, margarine, mayonnaise, salad dressing, sour cream, cheese, and cream cheese. Replace with low- or nonfat versions.
- Sauté with "Pam," water, wine, citrus juice (orange, lemon, lime), tomato juice, salsa, or broth.
- Choose nonfat or 1% dairy products.
- Low-fat snack ideas are fresh fruits and vegetables; nonfat or "light" yogurt, string cheese, low-fat lunch meats, whole-grain crackers, rice cakes, light popcorn, graham crackers, and pretzels. Keep in mind that many of these foods may contain carbohydrate.

4–2 ESTIMATING PORTION SIZES

Fist = 1 cup

Example: two servings of pasta or oatmeal

Palm = 3 oz.

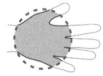

Example: a cooked serving of meat

Thumb Tip = 1 teaspoon

Example: a serving of mayonnaise or margarine

Handful = 1 or 2 oz. snack food

Example: 1 oz. nuts = 1 handful;
        2 oz. pretzels = 2 handfuls

Thumb = 1 oz.

Example: a piece of cheese

4–3 WEIGHT LOSS TIPS

We all have habits that need to change if we want to achieve and maintain a reasonable weight. Here is a list of ideas that may help you lose weight initially and then maintain your new weight:

- **Keep a food record.** Record the time, place, amount, and type of food you eat. Patterns of overeating and snacking will become obvious. Also, if you know you have to write it down, you may think twice about eating it.
- **Never go shopping at the supermarket when you are hungry.** You may be tempted to buy foods that you don't need and/or shouldn't eat. Take a shopping list—and stick to it!
- **Use smaller plates and dishes.** Smaller plates will make portions look larger and will have the psychological effect of making you feel fuller after eating.
- **Drink an 8-oz. glass of water before you begin your meal.** It will help take the edge off your appetite.
- **Eat slowly.** Savor each bite of food.
- **Eat all your meals in one location.** This will reduce the number of places you associate with food and eating.
- **Keep serving dishes in the kitchen.** You will be less likely to take second portions when the food is out of sight.
- **Put away leftovers before you start eating.** Save them for lunch the next day or freeze them for another meal. Store leftovers in covered bowls and containers—if they are not readily visible when the refrigerator is opened, you will be less likely to snack on them.
- **Avoid distractions while eating like watching television or reading.** Increased concentration on eating a meal will lead to increased satisfaction with the meal.
- **Eat before attending social functions that feature food.** It will help take the edge off your hunger and reduce the temptation to eat high-calorie foods.

Scripps Whittier Diabetes Institute

- **Never skip a meal.** It could be dangerous if you are taking diabetes medication or insulin—resulting in hypoglycemia (low blood glucose). Besides, most people find that skipping a meal generally leads to overeating at the next meal.
- **Set reasonable goals for yourself.** Weight reduction should be a slow process. You've had all your life to form bad habits and put the extra weight on—don't expect to change your habits and/or drop the extra weight overnight. Your goal is long-term weight management, not quick (and temporary) weight loss.
- **Don't weigh yourself too often.** It's easy to get discouraged when your weight doesn't change as much as you want. Hang in there—if you're eating less, you will see the results! Weigh yourself once a week and keep a record.
- **Reward your success with nonfood presents.** A new outfit, a new book, a mini-vacation, or something else to make you feel special.
- **Take up a new hobby instead of eating.** Family projects or community activities, for example. Many people eat from boredom and will find that other activities are much more satisfying.
- **Become more physically active.** Take a walk or do some other kind of exercise instead of eating. Contrary to popular belief, exercise does not increase hunger. It has the added advantage of burning calories and decreasing insulin needs. It also makes you feel good about yourself.
- **Make sure that you get the support you need to lose weight.** Family, friends, and support groups should help you to succeed.

4–4 What Are the Sources of Carbohydrates in the Diet?

The total amount of carbohydrate eaten rather than the type of carbohydrate has the greatest impact on your blood glucose.

Carbohydrate sources include simple or refined sources as well as complex carbohydrates (see examples below). Food sources of carbohydrate include starches and grains, fruits, fruit juices, dairy foods like milk and yogurt, sweets, sugar, and sweetened beverages.

Types of Carbohydrate

Simple or refined carbohydrates (processed, little fiber):

- All forms of sugar, white-flour products, and foods that have been highly processed
- Examples: Most pastas, white bread, white rice, instant mashed potatoes, bagels, fruit and vegetable juices, sugars, syrups, jams, honey, cookies, candy, sodas, milk, yogurt, processed cereals, and grain products

Complex carbohydrates (more fiber):

- Whole foods in their natural state such as whole grains, fresh fruits and vegetables, and legumes
- Examples: Whole wheat and whole-grain bread, brown and wild rice, whole potato, yams, sweet potatoes, whole-grain cereals, vegetables, cooked dried beans, peas, and lentils

Noncarbohydrate Foods (do not significantly affect your blood glucose)

Protein foods:

- Examples: Meat, poultry, fish, cheese, eggs, tofu, nut butters

Fats:
- Examples: Margarine, oil, mayonnaise, salad dressing, avocado, olives
- Be sure to check labels for carbohydrates, especially lower fat or nonfat sources because they may contain significant carbohydrates

4–5 SAMPLE MENU 1

1,500 Calories (1,600 Calories with Snack)

This calorie level is for most average-weight women and for men needing weight reduction. Use it as a temporary guide until a registered dietitian can assist you in personalizing your meal plan.

BREAKFAST

FOOD GROUP & SERVING SIZE:

Carbohydrates	(4 total = 60 g carbohydrate)	
Starch	2	1 100% whole wheat English muffin
Fruit	1	½ large banana
Milk	1	1 cup nonfat or 1% low-fat milk
Meat/Protein	1	1 slice (1 oz.) non/low-fat cheese
Fat	1	1 Tbsp. light margarine
Free Food		Coffee

LUNCH

FOOD GROUP & SERVING SIZE:

Carbohydrates	(4 total = 60 g carbohydrate)	
Starch	3	12" soft tortilla and ½ cup pinto beans
Fruit	1	1 cup small cantaloupe
Meat/Protein	2	(2 oz.) chicken breast
Vegetable	1	Chopped onion, tomato, and salsa
Fat	1	1 Tbsp. Ranch salad dressing
Free Food		Iced tea with lemon

DINNER

FOOD GROUP & SERVING SIZE:

Carbohydrates	(3 total = 45 g carbohydrate)	
Starch	2	1 100% whole-grain roll
		1 cup steamed red potatoes
Fruit	1	¾ cup fresh pineapple
Meat/Protein	3	3 oz. lean pork loin/chop

Vegetable	2	Green salad and ½ cup broccoli
Fat	1	1 Tbsp. light margarine or salad dressing
Free Food		½ cup sugar-free gelatin

EVENING SNACK*

FOOD GROUP & SERVING SIZE:

Starch *or* Fruit *or* Milk	1 (15 g carb.)	3 graham cracker squares or 1 apple or 1 carton (6–8 oz.) nonfat, low-fat, or light yogurt (i.e., Dannon Light)
Protein	1	¼ cup nonfat cottage cheese

Note: Necessary only if evening insulin is required.

4–6 SAMPLE MENU 2

1,500 Calories (1,600 Calories with Snack)

BREAKFAST

FOOD GROUP & SERVING SIZE:

Carbohydrates (4 total = 60 g carbohydrate)

Starch	2	2 slices 100% whole wheat toast
Fruit	1	1 small orange
Milk	1	1 cup nonfat or 1% low-fat milk
Meat/Protein	1	1 poached egg or ¼ cup egg substitute
Fat	1	1 Tbsp. light margarine
Free Food		Coffee

LUNCH

FOOD GROUP & SERVING SIZE:

Carbohydrates (4 total = 60 g carbohydrate)

Starch	3	6" submarine sandwich on 100% whole wheat bread 1 cup vegetable soup
Fruit	1	1 small pear
Meat/Protein	2	(1 oz.) Turkey & (1 oz.) low-fat cheese (on sandwich)
Vegetable	1	Lettuce, tomato, onion, pepper, etc.
Fat	1	1 Tbsp. light mayonnaise
Free Food		Diet soft drink, mustard, dill pickle

DINNER

FOOD GROUP & SERVING SIZE:

Carbohydrates (3 total = 45 g carbohydrate)

Starch	2	⅔ cup wild rice
Fruit	1	1 cup berries
Meat/Protein	3	3 oz. broiled lemon pepper white fish

⊃ Scripps Whittier Diabetes Institute

Vegetable	2	Green salad
		½ cup steamed zucchini
Fat	1	1 Tbsp. salad dressing
Free Food		Crystal Light beverage

EVENING SNACK*

FOOD GROUP & SERVING SIZE:

Starch *or* Fruit *or* Milk	1 (15 g carb.)	4–5 low-fat crackers or 1 cup berries or 1 cup nonfat or 1% low-fat milk
Protein	1	1 oz. string cheese

Note: Necessary only if evening insulin is required.

4–7 SAMPLE MENU 1

1,800 Calories (2,000 Calories with Snack)

This calorie level is for most average-weight men. Use it as a temporary guide until a registered dietitian can assist you in personalizing your meal plan.

BREAKFAST

FOOD GROUP & SERVING SIZE:

Carbohydrates	(4 total = 60 g carbohydrate)	
Starch	2	1 whole-grain English muffin
Fruit	1	½ large banana
Milk	1	1 cup nonfat or 1% low-fat milk
Meat/Protein	2	1 slice (1 oz.) non/low-fat cheese and ¼ cup egg substitute
Fat	1	1 Tbsp. light margarine
Free Food		Coffee

LUNCH

FOOD GROUP & SERVING SIZE:

Carbohydrates	(4 total = 60 g carbohydrate)	
Starch	3	12" soft whole wheat tortilla and ½ cup pinto beans
Fruit	1	1 cup cantaloupe
Meat/Protein	3	(3 oz.) chicken breast
Vegetable	1	Chopped onion, tomato, and salsa
Fat	1	1 Tbsp. Ranch salad dressing
Free Food		Iced tea with lemon

DINNER

FOOD GROUP & SERVING SIZE:

Carbohydrates	(4 total = 60 g carbohydrate)	
Starch	3	1 small 100% whole wheat roll
		1 cup steamed red potatoes
Fruit	1	¾ cup fresh pineapple

Meat/Protein	3	3 oz. lean pork loin/chop
Vegetable	2	Green salad and ½ cup green beans
Fat	2	1 Tbsp. each, light margarine and salad dressing
Free Food		½ cup sugar-free gelatin

EVENING SNACK*

FOOD GROUP & SERVING SIZE:

| Starch *or* Fruit *or* Milk | 1 (15 g carb.) | 3 graham cracker squares or ½ banana or 1 carton (6 to 8 oz.) non- or low-fat, light yogurt (i.e., Dannon Light) |
| Protein | 1 | ¼ cup nonfat cottage cheese or 1 oz. string cheese |

Note: Necessary only if evening insulin is required.

Scripps Whittier
Diabetes Institute

©2009

4–8 SAMPLE MENU 2

1,800 Calories (2,000 Calories with Snack)

BREAKFAST

FOOD GROUP & SERVING SIZE:

Carbohydrates	(4 total = 60 g carbohydrate)	
Starch	2	2 slices 100% whole-grain toast
Fruit	1	1 small orange
Milk	1	1 cup nonfat or 1% low-fat milk
Meat/Protein	2	2 poached eggs
Fat	1	1 Tbsp. light margarine
Free Food		Coffee

LUNCH

FOOD GROUP & SERVING SIZE:

Carbohydrates	(4 total = 60 g carbohydrate)	
Starch	3	6" submarine sandwich on whole wheat bread
		1 cup vegetable soup
Fruit	1	1 small pear
Meat/Protein	3	(2 oz.) Turkey & (1 oz.) low-fat cheese (on sandwich)
Vegetable	1	Lettuce, tomato, onion, pepper, etc.
Fat	1	1 Tbsp. light mayonnaise
Free Food		Diet soft drink, mustard, dill pickle

DINNER

FOOD GROUP & SERVING SIZE:

Carbohydrates	(4 total = 60 g carbohydrate)	
Starch	3	⅔ cup wild rice
		1 small whole-grain roll
Fruit	1	1 cup berries
Meat/Protein	3	3 oz. broiled lemon pepper whitefish
Vegetable	2	Green salad and 1 cup broccoli

Scripps Whittier Diabetes Institute

| Fat | 2 | 1 Tbsp. each, salad dressing and light margarine |
| Free Food | | Crystal Light beverage |

EVENING SNACK*

FOOD GROUP & SERVING SIZE:

| Starch *or* Fruit *or* Milk | 1 (15 g carb.) | 4–5 low-fat crackers or 1 cup melon or 1 cup nonfat or 1% low-fat milk |
| Protein | 1 | 1 oz. string cheese or ¼ cup nonfat cottage cheese |

*Note: Necessary only if evening insulin is required.

4–9 MAKE YOUR PLATE LOOK LIKE THIS!

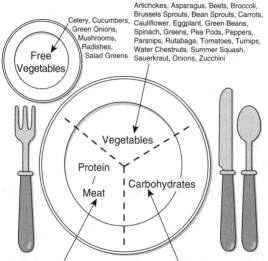

Free Vegetables

Celery, Cucumbers, Green Onions, Mushrooms, Radishes, Salad Greens

Artichokes, Asparagus, Beets, Broccoli, Brussels Sprouts, Bean Sprouts, Carrots, Cauliflower, Eggplant, Green Beans, Spinach, Greens, Pea Pods, Peppers, Parsnips, Rutabaga, Tomatoes, Turnips, Water Chestnuts, Summer Squash, Sauerkraut, Onions, Zucchini

Vegetables

Protein

Meat

Carbohydrates

Poultry (Chicken, Turkey) no skin, Fish, Lean Cuts of Beef, Pork, Lamb, Veal (trim fat and Bake, Broil, Boil or BBQ), Low-fat Cheese, Eggs, Egg Substitutes, Peanut Butter, Tofu, Low-fat Cottage Cheese, Other Nut Butters, Edameme

Fruit (fresh, canned in juice), Fat-free or 1% Milk, Plain or Light Yogurt, Whole Grain Bread, Tortillas, Rolls, English Muffins, Bagels, Crackers, Waffles, Pancakes, Muffin, Pita, Hamburger and Hot Dog Buns, Potato, Rice, Couscous, Pasta, Noodles, Corn, Peas, Sweet Potato, Lima Beans, Soybeans, Dried Peas and Beans (Pinto, Kidney, Garbanzo), Lentils, Winter Squash

> For weight control, fats should be used sparingly (e.g., margarine, oil, mayonnaise, salad dressing, gravy, sour cream, cream cheese, avocado, seeds, nuts, olives). Preferred fats are trans fat free.

4–10 MAKE YOUR PLATE LOOK LIKE THIS FOR WEIGHT CONTROL!

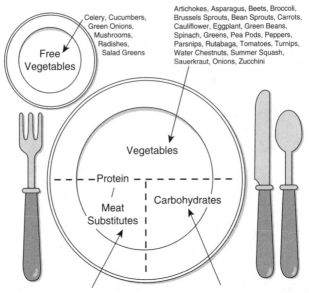

Free Vegetables: Celery, Cucumbers, Green Onions, Mushrooms, Radishes, Salad Greens

Artichokes, Asparagus, Beets, Broccoli, Brussels Sprouts, Bean Sprouts, Carrots, Cauliflower, Eggplant, Green Beans, Spinach, Greens, Pea Pods, Peppers, Parsnips, Rutabaga, Tomatoes, Turnips, Water Chestnuts, Summer Squash, Sauerkraut, Onions, Zucchini

Protein / Meat Substitutes: Poultry (Chicken, Turkey) no skin, Fish, Lean Cuts of Beef, Pork, Lamb, Veal (trim fat and Bake, Broil, Boil or BBQ), Low-fat Cheese, Eggs, Egg Substitutes, Peanut Butter, Tofu, Low-fat Cottage Cheese, Other Nut Butters, Edameme

Carbohydrates: Fruit (fresh, canned in juice), Fat-free or 1% Milk, Plain or Light Yogurt, Whole Grain Bread, Tortillas, Rolls, English Muffins, Bagels, Crackers, Waffles, Pancakes, Muffin, Pita, Hamburger and Hot Dog Buns, Potato, Rice, Couscous, Pasta, Noodles, Corn, Peas, Sweet Potato, Lima Beans, Soybeans, Dried Peas and Beans, (Pinto, Kidney, Garbanzo), Lentils, Winter Squash

> For weight control, fats should be used sparingly (e.g., margarine, oil, mayonnaise, salad dressing, gravy, sour cream, cream cheese, avocado, seeds, nuts, olives). Preferred fats are trans fat free.

Scripps Whittier Diabetes Institute

4–11 FOOD GROUPS AND SERVING SIZES

Carbohydrate Choices

FRUIT	STARCHES/BREAD	DAIRY
Apple, 1 small, 4 oz.	Bagel, ¼ of lg., ½ med	Buttermilk, low-fat,
Apricots, fresh, 4	(check label)	nonfat, 1 cup
Applesauce,	Barley, ⅓ cup	Evaporated, skim milk,
unsweetened,	Beans, peas, lentils, corn,	½ cup
½ cup	cooked, ½ cup	Nonfat yogurt, plain or
Banana, 1 small, 4 oz.,	Biscuit,* 2½" dia.	light, 6 oz.
or ½ large	Bread, 1 oz. slice	Nonfat milk, 1 cup
Berries, 1 cup	(check label)	1% Milk, 1 cup
Cantaloupe, ⅓ small	Bun, hot dog or	Soy milk, low-fat or
Canned fruit in own syrup	hamburger, ½ (1 oz.)	fat-free, 1 cup
drained, ½ cup	Cereal, cold flaked	
Dried fruit (check label)	(check label)	
Figs, fresh, 2 medium	Cereal, cooked, ½ cup	**Other carbohydrates:**
Grapefruit, ½ large	Couscous, ½ cup	Ice cream, light, no sugar
Grapes or Cherries,	Crackers, 4–5	added, ½ cup
6–10 large or 12–18	English muffin, ½	Pudding, sugar-free,
each, small, 3 oz.	Graham crackers, 3 squares	½ cup
Juice (100% fruit),	Melba toast, 5 slices	Soup, cream type, 1 cup
3–4 oz. (check label)	Pancake,* 1, 4" across	
Kiwi, 1 large	Pasta, cooked, ⅓ cup	
Mango, ½ large or ½ cup	Pita bread, ½, 6" across	
Melon, 1 cup	Popcorn, no added fat, 3 cups	
Mixed fresh fruit, 1 cup	Potato, 1 small (3 oz.)	
Nectarine, 1 medium	Potato, mashed, ½ cup	
Orange, 1 small, 6–½ oz.	Pretzels, ¾ oz.	
Papaya cubes, 1 cup	Rice, brown, wild or white,	
Peach, 1 medium	cooked, ⅓ cup	
Pear, ½ large	Squash, winter, 1 cup	1 cup = 8 oz.
Pineapple, fresh, ¾ cup	Sweet potato or yam, ½ cup	
Pineapple, canned, ½ cup	Tortilla, 6" across	
Plums, 2 small	Waffle, 4" square	
Prunes, dried, 3	Whole-grain bread,	
Raisins, 2 Tbsp.	1 slice (1 oz.) (check label)	
Tangerine, 2 small		
	*Includes 1 fat serving	
1 Choice =	1 Choice =	1 Choice =
15 g Carbohydrate	15 g Carbohydrate	15 g Carbohydrate
60 Calories	80–125 Calories	90–150 Calories

(continued)

Noncarbohydrate Choices

Fat	Meat/Protein	Vegetables
Monounsaturated	Beef (sirloin, round, ground round, flank, rump, tenderloin, lean)	Vegetables, cooked, ½ cup
Olive, Canola, Peanut oil, 1 tsp.		Vegetables, raw, 1 cup
Avocado, 2 Tbsp. or ⅛	Canadian Bacon	**For example:**
Nuts: Almonds, Cashews, 6	Fish (Halibut, Sea bass, Tilapia, Snapper, Mahi Mahi)	Artichoke / Mixed vegetables
Macadamia, 3		Asparagus / (without
Peanuts, 10		Beets / corn, peas,
Pecan halves, 4	Ham, lean	Broccoli / or pasta)
Natural peanut butter, ½ Tbsp.	Lamb (leg, chops, roast)	Brussels Sprouts / Mushrooms
Olives, 8–10 large	Luncheon meat, 98% fat-free	Cabbage / Okra
Tahini or Sesame paste, 2 tsp.	Pork (loin, tenderloin)	Carrots / Onions
		Cauliflower / Pea pods
Polyunsaturated	Poultry, no skin (chicken, turkey)	Celery / Peppers
Corn, Flaxseed, Safflower, Soy, Sunflower, Sesame oil, 1 tsp.	Seafood	Cucumbers / Radishes
	Veal (lean chop, roast)	Eggplant / Salad greens
		Green beans / (lettuce)
	Cheese	Greens / Sauerkraut
Margarine, tub or square, 1 tsp.	Cottage cheese, low-fat, ¼ cup	(collards, / Spinach
Margarine, Lite, 1 Tbsp.	Cheese, nonfat or low-fat, 1 oz.	kale, / Tomatoes
Salad dressing, 1 Tbsp.	Parmesan cheese, grated, 2 Tbsp.	mustard, / Turnips
Salad dressing, reduced fat, 2 Tbsp.		spinach, / Water
Mayonnaise, 1 tsp.		turnip) / Chestnuts
Mayonnaise, reduced fat, 1 Tbsp.	**Other**	Zucchini
Miracle Whip, 2 tsp.	Egg, 1 (up to 3 yolks/week)	**Note: Corn, peas, beans, lentils, and potatoes are listed under Starches/Bread**
Seeds: Pumpkin, Sunflower, 1 Tbsp.	Egg substitute, ¼ cup	1 cup = 8 oz.
Walnuts, 4 halves	Egg whites, 2	

Saturated and Trans Fat	Almond, Peanut, Cashew (natural) Butter,* 2 Tbsp.	If you eat 3 cups or more of raw vegetables or 1½ cups of cooked vegetables at one meal, count them as 1 carbohydrate choice (15 g carbohydrate).
Bacon, 1 strip	Tofu, light, 4 oz. or ½ cup	
Butter, stick, 1 tsp.	Tuna, packed in water, ¼ cup (1 oz.)	
Coconut milk, 1 Tbsp.		
Cream, Half & Half, 2 Tbsp.	*Includes 2 additional fat servings	
Cream Cheese, 1 Tbsp.		
Cream Cheese, reduced fat, 1-½ Tbsp.		
Mayonnaise, 1 tsp.		
Margarine, stick, 1 tsp.		
Shortening, 1 tsp		
Sour cream, 2 Tbsp.		
Sour cream, reduced fat, 3 Tbsp.		
1 Choice =	1 Choice = 1 ounce	1 Choice =
0 g Carbohydrate	0 g Carbohydrate	5 g Carbohydrate
45 Calories	35–100 Calories	25 Calories

4–12 DIETARY FIBER CONTENT OF SELECTED FOOD

Dietary fiber is carbohydrates in plant food that are not digested and therefore do not contribute to raising the blood glucose level. Dietary fiber exists in two basic forms, soluble and insoluble. Dietary fiber may help slow down the postmeal blood glucose rise by slowing down the digestion and absorption processes.

A good goal to aim for is 25–35 grams of total dietary fiber daily.

Dietary Fiber Content of Selected Foods

GRAMS OF FIBER	FRUITS
3.7	Apple, with Skin
2.7	Banana
2.1	Cantaloupe, ½ medium
1.7	Dates, Chopped, ⅛ cup dry
1.6	Grapes, 1 cup
2.2	Nectarine
3.1	Orange
0.5	Orange Juice, 1 cup
1.7	Peach
3.4	Peaches, 1 cup sliced
4.0	Pear
1.0	Plum
1.8	Prunes, Dried, 10
2.0	Prunes, Dried, Cooked, 1 oz.
0.8	Raisins, ⅛ cup
1.7	Strawberries, ½ cup
0.8	Watermelon, Diced, 1 cup

*All values are for 1 medium-sized fruit unless otherwise indicated.

GRAMS OF FIBER	VEGETABLES
2.3	Broccoli, Cooked, Chopped, ½ cup
1.3	Broccoli, Chopped, ½ cup
3.4	Brussels Sprouts, Cooked, ½ cup
1.6	Carrots, Shredded, ½ cup
2.2	Carrot, 1 medium
1.7	Cauliflower, Cooked, ½ cup
1.0	Celery, Diced, ½ cup
0.7	Celery, 1 stalk
2.0	Corn, Cooked, ½ cup
0.4	Cucumber, ½ cup
1.6	French Fry, 1 small (2.5 oz.)
1.6	Green Beans, Cooked (Frozen), ½ cup
1.0	Iceberg Lettuce, 1 cup
4.4	Peas, Cooked (Frozen) ½ cup
0.9	Peppers, Chopped, ½ cup
4.8	Potato, Baked with Skin
2.3	Potato, Baked without Skin
2.1	Potatoes, Mashed, ½ cup
1.3	Romaine lettuce, 1 cup
0.8	Spinach, ½ cup
2.8	Spinach, Cooked (Frozen), ½ cup
3.4	Sweet potato, Baked with Skin
0.3	Tomato, 1 slice
1.0	Tomato, 1 medium

*All values are for raw, uncooked vegetables unless otherwise indicated.

Scripps Whittier Diabetes Institute

(continued)

Grams of Fiber	Grains, Beans, And Nuts
7.5	Black Beans, ½ cup
2.5	Bran Muffin, 1 medium
5.3	Chickpeas, ½ cup
14.0	General Mills Fiber One, ½ cup
5.5	Kellogg's 40% Bran Flakes, 1 cup
0.7	Kellogg's Corn Flakes, 1 cup
7.3	Kidney Beans, ½ cup
7.8	Lentils, ½ cup
5.8	Lima Beans, ½ cup
4.0	Oatmeal, Cooked, 1 cup
5.8	Peanuts, ½ cup
1.9	Peanut Butter, Smooth, 2 Tbsp.
2.1	Peanut Butter, Chunky, 2 Tbsp.
0.7	Popcorn, Air-Popped, 1 cup
0.6	Rice, White, Cooked, 1 cup
2.0	Rice, Brown, Cooked, 1 cup
1.0	Sesame Seeds, 2 Tbsp.
1.2	Spaghetti, Cooked, ½ cup
1.1	Spinach Pasta, Cooked, ½ cup
1.5	Sunflower Seeds, ⅛ cup
0.6	Tortilla Chips, 1 cup (1.5 oz.)
1.6	Walnuts, Chopped, ¼ cup
7.6	Wheat Germ, ½ cup
0.6	Bread, White, 1 slice (1 oz.)
1.5	Bread, Whole Wheat, 1 slice (1 oz.)

*All values are for canned or cooked beans.

Source: Tufts University Diet and Nutrition Letter, 1995.

4–13 FAT FACTS

Saturated Fats

Stimulate your liver to produce more serum (blood) cholesterol. Saturated fats are found in two areas:

- Animal Fats: Butter, cream, lard, cheese, sour cream, whole and 2% milk, poultry skin, hot dogs, bacon, ribs, sausage, luncheon meats, and fatty cuts of red meats are some examples.
- Naturally Occurring Tropical Oils: Coconut oil, coconut milk, palm oil, palm kernel oil. Used predominately by the snack food industry.

Trans Fats

Also stimulate the liver to produce cholesterol. It is used heavily by food manufacturers in processed foods.

- On labels, they are listed under total fat.
- Hydrogenated Fats: Stick and tub margarine, vegetable shortening. Look for the term "partially hydrogenated oil" in the ingredient list, often in desserts.

Unsaturated Fats

Have been shown to decrease cholesterol if used to replace saturated fats. They are found in three areas:

- Monounsaturated Fats: Canola, peanut, and olive oils, avocado, olives, and most nuts (almonds, pecans, peanuts, hazelnuts, macadamias, pistachios).
- Polyunsaturated Fats: Soybean, cottonseed, sunflower, safflower, sesame, and corn oils; also walnuts.
- Omega-3 Fatty Acids: Cold-water fish (salmon, trout, cod, swordfish, herring, sardines, tuna, mackerel, anchovies), fish oil capsules, flax (seed, powder, oil), canola oil, soybeans and soybean oil, pumpkin seeds and pumpkin seed oil, walnuts and walnut oil, wheat germ.

4–14 Alcohol and Diabetes

Drinking too much alcohol is dangerous for everyone. As a person with diabetes, you should also **be aware that alcohol can cause hypoglycemia (low blood glucose),** especially if consumed without food.

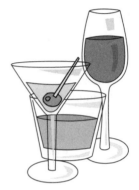

Alcohol can also be high in calories. If you choose to drink an occasional alcoholic beverage, you can usually do so safely *if* simple guidelines are followed:

- Check with your doctor prior to drinking alcohol. If alcohol is allowed for you—use **only in moderation.**
- Moderation is considered 1 serving a day for women and 2 servings a day for men.
- One serving of alcohol = 12 oz. of light beer, *or*
  = 1½ oz. of hard liquor, *or*
  = 5 oz. of dry wine

Caution:

- Alcohol can cause low blood sugar from 6 to 36 hours after its consumption, and the chance of low blood sugar is high in someone who eats minimally during the day and has a drink before or with dinner.
- Drink alcohol *only* with a meal or snack. Alcohol can cause low blood glucose. **Do not drink on an empty stomach!**
- If you are trying to lose weight, alcohol can add unnecessary calories.
- Avoid sweet wines, liqueurs, and sweetened mixed drinks because of the high sugar content. Acceptable mixers are diet carbonated beverages, club soda, mineral water, and diet tonic.
- Alcohol may be contraindicated with certain oral medications. Check with your doctor or a pharmacist.

4–15 Your Body Mass Index (BMI)

Find Your BMI

1. Find your height along the side of the chart.
2. Find your weight along the top of the chart.
3. Find the number in the box where your height meets your weight. This is your BMI.

Weight (pounds)

Height (feet/inches)	120	130	140	150	160	170	180	190	200	210	220	230	240	250	260	270	280	290	300	310	320	330
4'5"	30	33	35	38	40	43	45	48	50	53	55	58	60	63	65	68	70	73	75	78	80	83
4'6"	29	31	34	36	39	41	43	46	48	51	53	56	58	60	63	65	68	70	72	75	77	80
4'7"	28	30	33	35	37	40	42	44	47	49	51	54	56	58	61	63	65	68	70	72	75	77
4'8"	27	29	31	34	36	38	40	43	45	47	49	52	54	56	58	61	63	65	67	70	72	74
4'9"	26	28	30	33	35	37	39	41	43	46	48	50	52	54	56	59	61	63	65	67	69	72
4'10"	25	27	29	31	34	36	38	40	42	44	46	48	50	52	54	57	59	61	63	65	67	69
4'11"	24	26	28	30	32	34	36	38	40	43	45	47	49	51	53	55	57	59	61	63	65	67
5'0"	23	25	27	29	31	33	35	37	39	41	43	45	47	49	51	53	55	57	59	61	63	65
5'1"	23	25	27	28	30	32	34	36	38	40	42	44	45	47	49	51	53	55	57	59	61	62
5'2"	22	24	26	27	29	31	33	35	37	38	40	42	44	46	48	49	51	53	55	57	59	60
5'3"	21	23	25	27	28	30	32	34	36	37	39	41	43	44	46	48	50	51	53	55	57	59
5'4"	21	22	24	26	28	29	31	33	34	36	38	40	41	43	45	46	48	50	52	53	55	57
5'5"	20	22	23	25	27	28	30	32	33	35	37	38	40	42	43	45	47	48	50	52	53	55
5'6"	19	21	23	24	26	27	29	31	32	34	36	37	39	40	42	44	45	47	49	50	52	53
5'7"	19	20	22	24	25	27	28	30	31	33	35	36	38	39	41	42	44	46	47	49	50	52
5'8"	18	20	21	23	24	26	27	29	30	32	34	35	37	38	40	41	43	44	46	47	49	50
5'9"	18	19	21	22	24	25	27	28	30	31	33	34	36	37	38	40	41	43	44	46	47	49
5'10"	17	19	20	22	23	24	26	27	29	30	32	33	35	36	37	39	40	42	43	45	46	47
5'11"	17	18	20	21	22	24	25	27	28	29	31	32	34	35	36	38	39	41	42	43	45	46
6'0"	16	18	19	20	22	23	24	26	27	29	30	31	33	34	35	37	38	39	41	42	43	45
6'1"	16	17	19	20	21	22	24	25	26	28	29	30	32	33	34	36	37	38	40	41	42	44
6'2"	15	17	18	19	21	22	23	24	26	27	28	30	31	32	33	35	36	37	39	40	41	42
6'3"	15	16	18	19	20	21	23	24	25	26	28	29	30	31	33	34	35	36	38	39	40	41
6'4"	15	16	17	18	19	21	22	23	24	26	27	28	29	30	32	33	34	35	37	38	39	40
6'5"	14	15	17	18	19	20	21	23	24	25	26	27	29	30	31	32	33	34	36	37	38	39
6'6"	14	15	16	17	19	20	21	22	23	24	25	27	28	29	30	32	33	34	35	36	37	38
6'7"	14	15	16	17	18	19	20	21	23	24	25	26	27	28	29	30	32	33	34	35	36	37
6'8"	13	14	15	17	18	19	20	21	22	23	24	25	26	28	29	30	31	32	33	34	35	36
6'9"	13	14	15	16	17	18	19	20	21	22	23	24	25	26	27	28	29	30	31	32	34	35
6'10"	13	14	15	16	17	18	19	20	21	22	23	24	25	26	27	28	29	30	31	32	34	35

Underweight	Less than 18
Healthy Weight	19–24
Overweight	25–29
Obese	Over 30
Extreme Obesity	Over 40

Scripps Whittier Diabetes Institute

4–16 THE DOS AND DON'TS OF EXERCISE

It is recommended that you have your physician's participation and a thorough physical examination before beginning an exercise program.

Your diabetes should be under control before starting an exercise program.

EXERCISE DOS

- Check blood glucose before and after exercise
- Exercise at a moderate level and progress slowly
- Know the signs and symptoms of hypoglycemia
- Wear diabetes identification
- Always carry a sugar source
- Exercise 10 to 15 minutes after a snack 20 to 60 minutes after a meal
- Exercise 3 to 6 times a week
- Always warm-up and cool-down
- Monitor exercise intensity
- Drink water to replace lost fluids
- To avoid foot problems, invest in good shoes and avoid cement surfaces if possible

EXERCISE DON'TS

- Don't exercise when you are not feeling well
- Don't exercise in extreme heat, cold, or humidity
- Don't inject insulin into an area that will be exercised
- STOP if unusual pain occurs
- Don't exercise during insulin peak times
- Don't exercise if blood glucose is 250 mg/dL or or ketones are present
- Don't drink alcoholic beverages before, during, or after exercise

If a Low Blood Glucose Reaction Occurs!

- STOP exercise
- Test blood glucose
- Treat as needed
- Retest blood glucose
- Contact your doctor if reactions continue

Scripps Whittier
Diabetes Institute

4–17 THE BENEFITS OF EXERCISE

- Increases energy levels
- Burns unwanted calories
- Improves quality of sleep
- Reduces risk of illness and injury
- May increase insulin sensitivity
- May increase levels of HDL "Good Cholesterol"

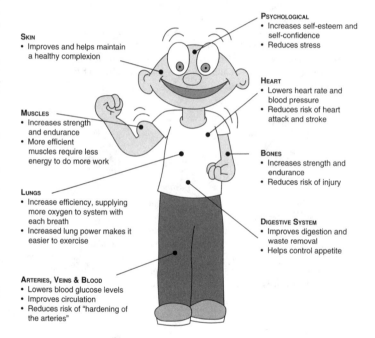

PSYCHOLOGICAL
- Increases self-esteem and self-confidence
- Reduces stress

SKIN
- Improves and helps maintain a healthy complexion

HEART
- Lowers heart rate and blood pressure
- Reduces risk of heart attack and stroke

MUSCLES
- Increases strength and endurance
- More efficient muscles require less energy to do more work

BONES
- Increases strength and endurance
- Reduces risk of injury

LUNGS
- Increase efficiency, supplying more oxygen to system with each breath
- Increased lung power makes it easier to exercise

DIGESTIVE SYSTEM
- Improves digestion and waste removal
- Helps control appetite

ARTERIES, VEINS & BLOOD
- Lowers blood glucose levels
- Improves circulation
- Reduces risk of "hardening of the arteries"

Scripps Whittier Diabetes Institute

4–18 Chair Exercises

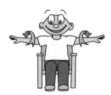

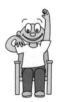

Arm Circles: Sit up straight in a chair. Keep your feet flat on the floor. Tuck in your tummy. Extend arms out to the sides at shoulder level. Make sure the elbows are straight. Circle the arms to the front 4 times. Then, circle the arms to the back 4 times. Gradually build up to 8 repetitions in each direction.

Hand Reaches: Sit in a chair. Place both hands on your shoulders. Extend your arm and reach toward the ceiling with your right hand. Return your right hand to your shoulder and repeat with your left hand. Gradually build up to 8 repetitions with each hand.

Lateral Stretch: Sit in a chair. Lift your right arm over your head and lean to the left. At the same time, make a C shape with your left arm (as if you were holding a baby). Gently stretch to the left. Change sides and repeat the exercise. Slowly build up to 8 repetitions on each side.

Marching in Place: Sit in a chair. Lift your left knee so that the foot is 6 inches off the floor. Lower your left knee. Lift your right knee so that the foot is 6 inches off the floor. Continue marching, lifting knees up and down.

Ankle Circles: Sit in a chair. Extend the right foot out in front. Circle the right ankle in 4 times. Circle the right ankle out 4 times. Repeat with the left foot.

Knee Pull: Sit in a chair. Pull your right knee into your chest. Hold the knee in for 4 seconds. Lower the leg. Repeat with the other knee.

Scripps Whittier Diabetes Institute

References

1. American Diabetes Association. Nutrition recommendations and interventions for diabetes. *Diabetes Care.* January 2008;31(suppl 1): s61–s78.

2. Beaser R. *Joslin's Diabetes Deskbook: A Guide for Primary Care Providers.* 2nd ed. Lippincott Williams & Wilkins and Joslin Diabetes Center; Philadelphia, PA, 2007:86.

3. American Diabetes Association. Dietary carbohydrate (amount and type) in the prevention and management of diabetes. *Diabetes Care.* 2004;27:2266–2271.

4. American Heart Association. Meat, poultry and fish. Available at: http://www.americanheart.org/presenter.jhtml?identifier=4627. Accessed October 27, 2009.

5. US Department of Health and Human Services, National Institutes of Health, National Heart, Lung, and Blood Institute. *Your Guide to Lowering Your Blood Pressure with DASH: DASH Eating Plan.* Available at: http://www.nhlbi.nih.gov/health/public/heart/hbp/dash/new_dash.pdf. Accessed October 27, 2009.

6. Anderson RA. Chromium glucose intolerance and diabetes. *J Am Coll Nutr.* 1998;17:548–555.

7. Sjogren A, Floren CH, Nilsson A. Magnesium, potassium and zinc deficiency in subjects with type II diabetes mellitus. *Acta Med Scand.* 1988;224:461–466. Available at: http://www.ncbi.nlm.nih.gov/pubmed/3202015. Accessed October 27, 2009.

8. Liu S. Dietary calcium, vitamin D and the prevalence of metabolic syndrome in middle-aged and older U.S. women. *Diabetes Care.* 2005;28:2926–2932.

9. Mayo Clinic. Dietary fiber: an essential part of a healthy diet. Available at: http://www.mayoclinic.com/health/fiber/nu00033/NSECTIONGROUP=2. Accessed October 27, 2009.

10. American Association of Diabetes Educators. *The Art and Science of Diabetes Self-Management Education: A Desk Reference for Healthcare Professionals.* Chicago, IL: American Association of Diabetes Educators; 2006:379.

11. Bode B. *Pumping Protocol: A Physician Guide to Insulin Pump Therapy Initiation.* 2008:13. Supported by an educational grant from MiniMed.

12. American Diabetes Association. Standards of medical care in diabetes—2009. *Diabetes Care.* 2009;32:s13–s61.

13. Colberg S. On the cutting edge. *DM Care and Educ.* Winter 2005–2006;26:19–23.

14. Walsh J, Roberts R, Roberts R. *Pumping Insulin.* 4th ed. San Diego, Calif: Torrey Pines Press; 2006.

5 ▪ Diabetes and Heart Disease Walk Hand in Hand: Goals for Glucose, Hypertension, and Dyslipidemia

It is notable that two out of three people with diabetes die from heart disease. The link between the two ailments is strong and significant, and a close eye should be kept on symptoms so that a diabetic patient—or anyone at risk for heart disease—does not become another statistic. At every turn, cardiovascular disease, especially cardiovascular death, stalks the patient with diabetes. When matching individuals with diabetes to nondiabetes in heart disease studies, those with diabetes have always fared worse.

Diabetes has garnered even more attention recently, particularly with the emergence of new data indicating that the risk of cardiovascular disease events in people with diabetes may be higher than once suspected. Recognizing its increased incidence and prevalence, researchers have focused on examining the correlation between diabetes and cardiovascular risk, ways to combat the disease, and a means by which to educate the public regarding the devastating effects of the disease.

The diabetic risks associated with heart disease include high blood pressure, high low-density lipoprotein (LDL) cholesterol, high triglycerides, low high-density lipoprotein (HDL) cholesterol, smoking, obesity, poorly controlled blood glucose levels, and lack of physical activity. Many more ailments exist that can affect many parts of the body and can lead to serious complications, including blindness, kidney disease, nervous system disease, periodontal disease, amputations, and complication of pregnancy, to name just a few.

Heart and Stroke Risk Factors for People with Diabetes

- High blood pressure
- Lipid disorders
- High LDL cholesterol
- High triglycerides
- Low HDL cholesterol
- Smoking
- Obesity
- Lack of physical activity
- Poorly controlled blood glucose

Controlling risk factors is the single most important way to suspend or even prevent the onset of cardiovascular disease and stroke in diabetes patients. Controlling glucose as a means of lowering the risk of cardiovascular disease has become controversial recently in light of the recently released ACCORD, ADVANCE, and VADT results.[1-3] Despite the results of these studies, which indicate that intensive glucose management had no greater benefit than conventional glucose control did or, with ACCORD, had worse outcomes, there are some key points to keep in mind that may help direct the decision on how tight to control blood glucose.

Studies such as the long-term outcomes of the EDIC study in type 1 diabetes demonstrate a 50% reduction in cardiovascular disease in the group that had been intensively controlled during the intervention period compared to the standard care group, and in the long-term follow-up of the UKPDS, there were significant differences in reduction of microvascular and macrovascular outcomes in the groups initially randomized to the intensively managed groups.[4-6]

The current recommendations of the American Diabetes Association are to target a HbA1c of less than 7% and to individualize this target based on the specific situation of each patient. It may be wise in older patients, with more advanced heart disease, to keep their HbA1c closer to 7–7.5% and in younger patients who are earlier in their diagnosis of diabetes to target a HbA1c lower than 7%. The added benefit of protection from microvascular disease can also be seen when optimizing a HbA1c level and a reduction by even one percentage point can reduce risk factors for retinal, renal, and neurologic diseases by 40–60%.

Keeping blood pressure in check can also reduce the risk of cardiovascular disease. In general, for every 10 mm Hg reduction in systolic blood pressure, the risk for complications related to diabetes is reduced by 12%.[7,8] Treatment with angiotensin-converting enzyme inhibitors and angiotensin receptor blockers remains the first choice for treatment in diabetes as long as there are no contraindications to using these agents, such as severe renal insufficiency, hyperkalemia, or cough.[9] Diuretics, calcium channel blockers, and beta blockers can be considered as alternative and additional choices, and selection of agents is dependent on other comorbid conditions, which may dictate the choice of agents. For example, for significant systolic hypertension, a diuretic and calcium channel blockers are good choices; for individuals with coronary disease, a beta blocker may be needed.

Improved control of blood lipids, or cholesterol, can reduce cardiovascular complications for a diabetic patient by 20–50%.[10] It is critical to reduce the LDL by 30% from baseline or below 100 mg/dL.[9] In patients with existing cardiovascular disease, an LDL of less than 70 mg/dL is recommended. Statins are the primary agent for treatment of dyslipidemia if dietary measures are not successful, and they have demonstrated significant benefits in numerous studies.[11–13] It remains unclear whether elevated triglycerides should be targeted for treatment in patients with diabetes.

The VA-HIT trial included patients with diabetes and pre-diabetes. Gemfibrozil was used as the primary treatment agent, and as a result triglycerides were significantly lowered with a minimal effect on LDL cholesterol. The VA-HIT study shows that gemfibrozil is extremely effective in reducing cardiovascular risk in people with features of the metabolic syndrome such as overweight, hypertriglyceridemia, and low HDL-C. This study demonstrates reduction in cardiovascular disease with the study population, but together with the Helsinki Heart Study it is the only study to date to clearly show this as a primary outcome.[14] Results from the nearly completed ACCORD study will evaluate whether adding fenofibrate to a statin in patients with type 2 diabetes will result in lowering cardiovascular disease. Until those results are released, the decision to treat with combination statin/fibrate in diabetes remains individualized and must be monitored carefully for any indications of myositis or renal insufficiency.

Additional agents that control cholesterol may be useful in diabetes but require special precautions. Resin binding agents such as cholestyramine and colestipol are very effective in lowering LDL but may increase triglyceride levels, which are already somewhat elevated in diabetes. Similar effects are seen with colesevelam (Welchol). Nicotinic acid in higher doses (above 1,500 mg per day) can lower LDL and triglycerides and raise HDL cholesterol. Although this profile may seem beneficial for the specific lipid pattern seen in diabetes, nicotinic acid also has an effect on worsening insulin resistance and may require monitoring and adjustment of glucose-lowering medications. Side effects of nicotinic acid such as flushing, rash, and liver enzyme elevations may also inhibit use of this agent. Most recently, ezetimibe (Zetia) has entered the market as an LDL-lowering agent. Although very effective as an LDL-lowering agent, especially in combination with a statin, it remains unclear what the effect on cardiovascular outcomes is. Several ongoing long-term trials using this agent will better guide healthcare providers in the future. At this time, the preferred methods of cholesterol control using lipid-lowering agents in diabetes are statins, and if LDL still is not controlled, the addition of resin binding agents or niacin can be considered. Ezetimibe can be added if these methods are not effective or contraindicated. Fibrates can be used to lower triglycerides, but patients must be monitored carefully for signs of myositis and renal insufficiency, especially if used in combination with statins.

Pre-diabetes is also an indicator that full-blown diabetes can be lurking just around the corner, and a swift and routine adjustment in diet and exercise can stave off the onset altogether. Unfortunately, individuals with pre-diabetes have an increased risk of developing type 2 diabetes, heart disease, and stroke. Pre-diabetes is a condition in which individuals have blood glucose levels higher than normal but not high enough to be classified as diabetes. Other pre-diabetes signs include an impaired fasting glucose or a condition in which the fasting blood sugar level is 100–125 mg/dL after an overnight fast. Impaired glucose tolerance is a condition in which the blood sugar level is 140–199 mg/dL after a 2-hr oral glucose tolerance test. Both conditions are not normal, but also not high enough to diagnose diabetes. Initiating treatment for lipid lowering and blood pressure lowering in this high-risk group of patients is imperative if their LDL cholesterol and blood pressure are not within target range (LDL <100 mg/dL and blood pressure <130/80 mm HG).

Achieving an ideal body weight and making sure blood pressure, cholesterol, and blood glucose levels are at the recommended targets are imperative. Currently, the recommendations of the American Diabetes Association for these levels are as follows:

1. Blood pressure less than 130/80 mm HG
2. LDL cholesterol less than 100 mg/dL
3. A1c less than 7%

In general for a healthy heart and to control sugar levels, it is important that individuals eat a nutritionally balanced diet rich in vegetables, fruits, lean proteins, and whole grains and minimize sweets and refined sugars as much as possible. The old adage holds true: "Eat, drink, and be merry," but individuals should do so in moderation, especially if there an increased risk of diabetes, heart disease, or stroke in their family.

Diabetes Resource Toolkit

Patient Education

5–1 Eat Less Salt

5–2 Sources of Cholesterol and Fat

5–3 Types of Fat in Blood

Clinical Resources

5–4 Classification of Hyperlipidemia

5–5 Lifestyle Modifications

5–6 HTN Management Program

5–1 Eat Less Salt

Sodium and salt are found in most foods. Sodium helps to control body fluids, but too much sodium or salt can be bad. Most of the sodium we eat comes from:

- Processed Foods: bacon, sausage, hot dogs, lunchmeats, cheese, chips, crackers, frozen dinners.

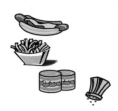

- Prepared Foods: fast food, restaurant food.
- Canned Foods: soups, vegetables, beans, pickles, meats.
- Seasonings: salt, soy sauce, steak sauce, seasoning blends, bouillon, fish sauce, salad dressing.

How much sodium is ok?

Try not to eat more than 2000–3000 mg of sodium each day.

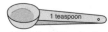

1 tsp salt = 2300 mg sodium

Why is too much sodium bad?

Too much sodium can cause high blood pressure (hypertension). High blood pressure can cause:

- Heart attack
- Stroke
- Eye problems
- Kidney/liver damage

Scripps Whittier
Diabetes Institute
©2009

To eat less sodium

Read food labels and look for the words salt and sodium.
Don't eat canned and pickled foods with more than 400 mg of
sodium a serving.

- Choose more of
  - Fresh or frozen vegetables and fruits
  - Salt-free or low sodium food
  - Low-fat dairy products (yogurt and milk)
- Eat less of
  - Snack foods
  - Processed cheese and meats
  - Fast food

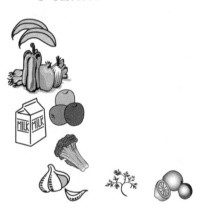

- Choose more of
  - Fresh herbs or garlic
  - Low sodium
    seasoning blends
  - Lemon juice and
    vinegar
- Use less of
  - Salt in recipes
  - Garlic/onion salt
  - Soy sauce
  - Steak sauce and
    meat tenderizers

Eat Less Salt
Translation of this publication was supported by HRSA HCAP Grant
G92OA02204.
©2006 The Whittier Institute for Diabetes

Permission granted by The Whittier Institute for Diabetes to copy
for patient education purposes. For additional information see www.
whittier.org

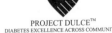

PROJECT DULCE™
DIABETES EXCELLENCE ACROSS COMMUNITIES

5–2 SOURCES OF CHOLESTEROL AND FAT

CHOLESTEROL (Limit These)	SATURATED/ TRANS FAT (Limit These)	UNSATURATED FAT	
Meat	Meat	Safflower oil	
Cheese	Cheese	Sunflower oil	
Egg yolk	Egg yolk	Corn oil	
Whole milk	Whole milk	Soybean oil	--Polyunsaturated
Reduced fat (2%) milk	Reduced-fat (2%) milk	Sesame oil	
Ice cream	Ice cream	Walnuts	
Butter	Cream cheese	Sesame seeds	
Organ meats	Sour cream		
Shellfish	Palm oil	Olive oil	
	Coconut oil	Canola oil	
	Hydrogenated or partially hydrogenated vegetable oil	Olives	
	Poultry with skin	Avocados	--Monounsaturated (choose more often)
	Margarine	Almonds	
		Cashews	
		Pecans	

5–3 Types of Fat in Blood

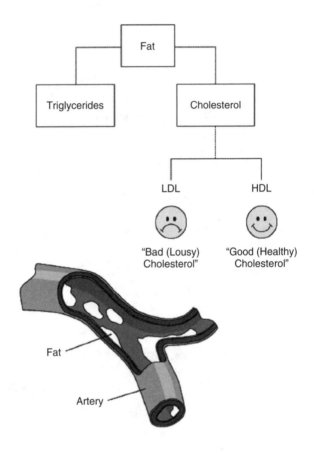

Lipid Management in Diabetes

5–4 CLASSIFICATION OF HYPERLIPIDEMIA

☐ **LDL above target** ☐ **LDL & TG above target** ☐ **HDL below target**

1. **Individualized lipid goal:** <100 (Except in certain
   circumstances such as overt CVD when a target of <70 mg/dL
   is an option)

   ☐ LDL <100 (all pts with DM and CAD) or
   ☐ LDL <70 (overt CVD) or
   ☐ 30–40% LDL reduction from baseline LDL
   ☐ HDL >40 men HDL >50 female
   ☐ T Chol <200
   ☐ TG <150

2. **Labs**

☐ Chemistry panel ☐ Fasting lipid profile ☐ Liver function tests (AST/ALT) ☐ TSH	Baseline labs should be within 3 months of initiating lipid drug therapy (**AST/ALT >3 × ULN lipid-lowering drug therapy may be contraindicated**) **Check CPK if symptoms of severe myalgia**

Lipid Management Program

This clinical guideline is designed to assist primary care providers
(PCPs) to individualize treatment plans and set goals for adult,
nonpregnant patients with hyperlipidemia and diabetes. This
guideline is not intended to replace sound medical judgment or
clinical decision making and may need to be adapted for special
populations.

After the PCP conducts a patient evaluation, including
history and physical, it is recommended that the patient

be referred to diabetes education for education. Lifestyle modifications are essential to lipid control. The diabetes team (RN, RD, peer educator) will address the following behavior/ lifestyle modification topics when applicable: weight reduction, physical activity, alcohol consumption, smoking cessation, stress, and medication adherence.

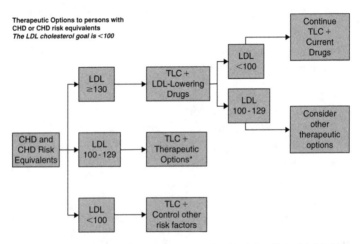

*Therapeutic options include LDL-lowering dietary or drug therapies, emphasizing weight reduction and increased physical activity, adding drugs to lower triglycerides or raise HDL cholesterol (nicotinic acid or fibrates), and intensifying control of other risk factors.

NCEP ATP II I Guidelines Update July 2004
ADA Clinical Practice Recommendations 2008
Staged Diabetes Management: Prevention, Detection and Treatment Diabetes in Adults. 4th Edition Revised

ADA 2009 Standards of Care have added the option of lowering LDL to <70 mg/dL in patients with overt CVD or lowering the LDL by 30–40% from baseline. This decision is individualized by the patient's PCP.

5–5 LIFESTYLE MODIFICATIONS

Modification	Recommenda-tions	Diabetes Education Team or Other Service Available	Systolic BP Reduction Ranges
Weight reduction	Maintain normal body weight (BMI <25)	Refer for Nutritional counseling RD, CDE—Classes Depression care manager RN, CD—education and monitoring	5–20 mm Hg/10-kg weight loss
Adopt DASH eating plan	Consume diet rich in fruits, vegetables, and low-fat diary products with a reduced content of saturated and total fat	Refer for Nutritional counseling RD, CDE—Classes RN, CDE—education and monitoring	8–14 mm Hg
Sodium restriction	Reduce dietary sodium intake to no more than 100 meEq/L (2.4 g sodium or 6 g sodium chloride)	Refer for Nutritional counseling RD, CDE—Classes RN, CDE case manager—education and monitoring	2–8 mm Hg
Physical activity	Engage in regular aerobic physical activity such as brisk walking (at least 30 minutes per day, most days of the week)	Classes RN, CDE—education and monitoring	4–9 mm Hg

(continued)

Moderation of alcohol consumption	Limit consumption to no more than 2 drinks/day for men and 1 drink/day for women and lighter persons	Refer for Nutritional counseling RD, CDE—Classes Depression care manager RN, CDE—education and monitoring	2–4 mm Hg
Smoking cessation	Tobacco cessation counseling or programs, nicotine patch/gum or medications	Refer to 1-800-NO-BUTTS Depression care manager RN, CDE—education and monitoring	Smoking cessation decreases risk of CV events
Verify adherence to medications	Assess at each visit, support patient with adherence to medication regimen considering above lifestyle modifications	Classes RN, CDE—education and monitoring RD, CDE reinforcement	Compliance increases likelihood of meeting goals
Psychosocial issues	Assess at initial and periodic visits factors such as anxiety/stress, depression, or other psychosocial issues	Depression manager or other clinical or mental health team member as assigned by the clinic or PCP	Not determined

5–6 HTN MANAGEMENT PROGRAM

This clinical guideline is designed to assist primary care providers (PCPs) to individualize treatment plans and set goals for adult, nonpregnant patients with hypertension with or without diabetes. This guideline is not intended to replace sound medical judgment or clinical decision making and may need to be adapted for special populations.

After the PCP conducts a diabetes evaluation, including history and physical, it is recommended that the patient be referred to a diabetes education program for education. Lifestyle modifications are essential to hypertension control. The diabetes education team (RN, RD, peer educator) can address the following behavior/lifestyle modification topics when applicable: weight reduction, physical activity, alcohol consumption, smoking cessation, stress, and medication adherence.

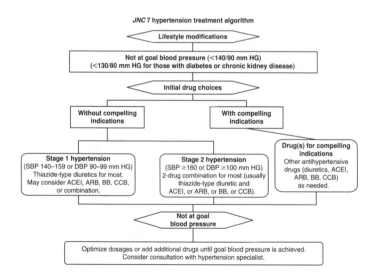

JNC 7 hypertension treatment algorithm

HTN with Compelling Indicators

Compelling Indicators	Recommended Diuretics	Drugs BB	ACE	ARB	CCB	Aldo ANT
Heart Failure	x	x	x	x		x
Postmyocardial Infarction		x	x			x
High CAD Disease Risk	x	x	x		x	
Diabetes	x	x	x	x	x	
Chronic Kidney Disease			x	x		
Recurrent Stroke Prevention	x		x			

Source: Adapted from: National Heart, Lung, and Blood Institute. *JNC 7 Express. The Seventh Report of the Joint National Committee on the Prevention, Detection, Evaluation and Treatment of High Blood Pressure.* 2003.

The Art and Science of Diabetes Self Management Education. American Association of Diabetes Educators; 1st ed., 2006.

Staged Diabetes Management: Prevention, Detection and Treatment of Diabetes in Adults. 4th ed. Revised.

References

1. Nathan DM, Cleary PA, Backlund JY, et al. Intensive diabetes treatment and cardiovascular disease in patients with type 1 diabetes. *N Engl J Med.* 2005;22:2643–2653.

2. ADVANCE Collaborative Group. Intensive blood glucose control and vascular outcomes in patients with type 2 diabetes. *N Engl J Med.* 2008;358:2560–2572.

3. ACCORD Study Group. Effects of intensive glucose lowering in type 2 diabetes. *N Engl J Med.* 2008;358:2545–2559.

4. Diabetes Control and Complications Trial Research Group. The effect of intensive treatment of diabetes on the development and progression of long-term complications of insulin-dependent diabetes mellitus. *N Engl J Med.* 1993;329:997–986.

5. UK Prospective Diabetes Study (UKPDS) Group. Intensive blood-glucose control with sulphonylureas or insulin compared with conventional treatment and risk of complications in patients with type 2 diabetes (UKPDS 33). *Lancet.* 1998;352:837–853.

6. Holman RR, Paul SK, Bethel MA, Matthews DR, Neil AW. 10-year follow-up of intensive glucose control in type 2 diabetes. *N Engl J Med.* 2008;359:1577–1589.

7. Adler AI, Stratton IM, Neil HA, et al. Association of systolic blood pressure with macrovascular and microvascular complications of type 2 diabetes (UKPDS 36): prospective observational study. *BMJ.* 2000;321(7258):412–419.

8. Stratton IM, Adler AI, Neil HA, et al. Association of glycaemia with macrovascular and microvascular complications of type 2 diabetes (UKPDS 35): prospective observational study. *BMJ.* 2000;321(7258):405–412.

9. American Diabetes Association. Standards of medical care in diabetes—2009. *Diabetes Care.* 2009;32:s13–s61.

10. Randomised trial of cholesterol lowering in 4444 patients with coronary heart disease: the Scandinavian Simvastatin Survival Study (4S). *Lancet.* November 19, 1994;344(8934):1383–1389.

11. LaRosa JC, Grundy SM, Waters DD, et al. Intensive lipid lowering with atorvastatin in patients with stable coronary disease. *N Engl J Med.* 2005;352:1425–1435.

12. Steinberg D, Glass CK, Witztum JL. Evidence mandating earlier and more aggressive treatment of hypercholesterolemia. *Circulation.* 2008;118:672–677.

13. Domanski MJ. Primary prevention of coronary artery disease. *N Engl J Med.* 2007;357:1543–1545.

14. Barter PJ, Rye KA. Is there a role for fibrates in the management of dyslipidemia in the metabolic syndrome? *Arteriosclr Thromb Vasc Biol.* 2008;28:39–46.

6 ■ Standards of Care and Prevention and Treatment of Microvascular and Macrovascular Complications

ADA Standards of Care

Table 6.1 lists the current American Diabetes Association standards of care for patients with diabetes.

Table 6.1	ADA Standards of Care		
TEST	FREQUENCY	GOAL	COMMENTS
A1c	Every 3 months. If A1c at goal, every 6 months.	<7%	The following may affect the A1c result: anemia, blood loss, chronic renal failure, episodes of severe hypoglycemia and hyperglycemia *Individualize A1c goals—patients with comorbid conditions, history of severe hypoglycemia, or limited life expectancy consider higher A1c goal
			ADA recommends using the verbiage "estimated average glucose" (e AG) when talking with patients instead of "A1c," which can be confusing to patients. A new glucose calculating formula that is similar to the formula used for glucose meters provides values that more closely correlate to the patient meter. See http://professional.diabetes. org/GlucoseCalculator.aspx for further detail.

(continued)

Table 6.1   ADA Standards of Care *(continued)*

TEST	FREQUENCY	GOAL	COMMENTS
Blood glucose monitoring in the home	Multiple daily insulin injections check at least 3 times a day. Oral agents, basal insulin, or diet and exercise suggest frequency to the patient based on current glucose status and risk factors for hypoglycemia.	Pre meal 70–130 mg/dL 2-hr post meal <180 mg/dL	Two-hour postprandial (begins at first bite) checks are valuable to assess the effects of food, bolus insulin doses, and some fast-acting oral agents.
BP	Every visit.	<130/80 mm Hg	Many patients require 3 or more antihypertensive medications to reach goal.
Lipids Cholesterol Triglycerides LDL HDL	Annually and as needed with medication changes.	C <200 mg/dL T <150 mg/dL LDL <100 mg/dL LDL* <70 mg/dL HDL♂ >40 mg/dL HDL♀ >50 mg/dL	*Lower LDL recommended for patients with overt CVD.
Urine microalbumin	Type 1 screen 5 years after diagnosis and type 2 at diagnosis, then yearly.	<30 normal Microalbuminuria 30 to 299 Macroalbuminuria (clinical) ≥300	
Glomerular filtration rate	Yearly	Stage 1 ≥90 Stage 2 60–89 Stage 3 30–59 Stage 4 15–29 Stage 5 <15 or dialysis GFR (mL/min per 1.73 m² body surface area)	GFR calculators are available at http://www.nkdep.nih.gov. Consult a nephrologist at stage 4 or sooner depending on individual patient status.
Aspirin therapy	Daily	75 mg to 162 mg/ day	Consider for high risk cardiovascular patients. Insufficient data to recommend as primary prevention for low risk persons. Clinical judgement required. Contraindicated in patients younger than

		age 21 years because of the associated risk of Reye's syndrome.
		For patients with CVD with a documented allergy to aspirin use clopidogrel 75 mg/day.
Foot exam	Every visit for visual inspection and yearly complete foot exam.	Complete foot exam includes • Tuning fork • 10-g monofilament • Hammer • Pinprick sensation • Pulses, skin, nails examination • Assessment for foot deformities • Patient daily self-examination at home is crucial to preventing foot ulcers
Smoking cessation	Every visit.	Free telephone quit lines are available in each state: www.naquitline.org.
Dental exam	Twice a year.	Smoking cessation, proper brushing and flossing.
Dilated eye exam	Type 1 screen 5 years after diagnosis and type 2 at diagnosis, then yearly for both.	Women with preexisting diabetes who are planning pregnancy or who have become pregnant should have a comprehensive eye examination and be counseled on the risk of development and/or progression of diabetic retinopathy.
RD visits	Once a year after initial education classes and as needed.	MNT, when delivered by a registered dietitian, is reimbursed as part of the Medicare program (www.cms.hhs.gov/medicalnutritiontherapy)
Diabetes Self-Management Education Classes (DSME)	At diagnosis and as needed thereafter.	DSME, when provided by an ADA ERP program, is reimbursed as part of the Medicare program (www.cms.hhs.gov/DiabetesSelfManagement).

(continued)

Table 6.1   ADA Standards of Care *(continued)*

TEST	FREQUENCY	GOAL	COMMENTS
			Studies have found that DSME is associated with improved diabetes knowledge, improved self-care behavior, improved clinical outcomes, and improved quality of life.
Flu shot	Yearly.		For all patients ≥6 months of age.
Pneumococcal vaccine	See comments.		Patients ≥2 years of age. A one-time revaccination is recommended for individuals >64 years of age previously immunized when they were <65 years of age if the vaccine was administered >5 years ago.
Family planning	Every visit with women of childbearing age.		Poor glucose control during conception leads to a higher risk of birth defects and spontaneous miscarriages.
Psychosocial assessment	Every visit.		Higher rates of depression.

Metabolic Goals to Reduce Complications

True or false: Diabetes is the leading cause of amputations, blindness, and renal failure?

The answer is false. *Uncontrolled diabetes* is the leading cause of amputations, blindness, and renal failure. Managing blood glucose, lipids, and blood pressure is critical to preventing complications from diabetes.

Table 6.2 lists the complications of diabetes. **Table 6.3** lists risk factors that contribute to complications of diabetes. And **Table 6.4** lists different methods of preventing and treating diabetic complications.

Table 6.2   Complications of Diabetes

Microvascular Disease	Macrovascular Disease
Nephropathy	Coronary artery disease
Retinopathy	Stroke
Neuropathy	Peripheral vascular disease
Dental disease	
▼	▼
Blood Glucose Management	Blood Pressure, Lipids Management
Other—sleep apnea	Other risk factors—smoking

Table 6.3   Risk Factors That Contribute to Complications of Diabetes

Risk Factors	Modifiable
Nonmodifiable	• Blood glucose
• Age	• Blood pressure
• Duration of diabetes	• Lipids
• Gender	• Platelets
• Race	• Homocystine levels
• Genetics	• Smoking
	• Nutrition
	• Weight
	• Exercise
	• Stress

Table 6.4   Prevention and Treatment of Diabetic Complications

	Prevention	Precautions	Treatment*	Comments
Nephropathy	Annual albumin and GFR screening, blood pressure and A1c control Smoking cessation	Risk of CVD is increased 1.4–2.05 times with creatinine >1.4–1.5 mg/dL.[†] Risk of CVD is increased 1.5–3.5 times with microalbuminuria. Monitor potassium serum and	Type 1 with any degree of albuminuria treat with an ACEI Type 2 with HTN and microalbuminuria both ACEI & ARBs are effective—if macroalbuminuria and serum Cr >1.5 mg/dL ARBs delay	African Americans 3.8× higher risk[†] Native Americans 2.0× Asians 1.3× Team with a nephrologist once the GFR is 30 mL/min/1.73 m^2 or less Renal disease as evidenced by albuminuria and ↑ serum Cr is a

(continued)

Table 6.4   Prevention and Treatment of Diabetic Complications *(continued)*

	PREVENTION	PRECAUTIONS	TREATMENT*	COMMENTS
		and creatinine with use of ACE, ARBs, and diuretics.	progression of nephropathy Diuretics, beta-blockers, and calcium channel blockers as additional therapy ↓ protein 0.8–1.0 g/kg in early stages CKD and ↓ 0.8 g/kg in late stages	predictor of retinopathy‡ See www.nkdep.nih.gov
Retinopathy	Annual dilated eye exam, blood pressure, A1c and lipid control, smoking cessation	No activity that requires heavy lifting or jarring head movements with moderate or severe retinopathy.‡	Laser photocoagulation therapy with macular edema and PDR and some severe cases of NPDR	Higher rate of cataracts and glaucoma with diabetes as well Up to 21% of people with type 2 will have some degree of retinopathy at diagnosis See American Optometric Association at www.aao.org See American Council for the Blind at www.acb.org
Neuropathy—most common form: distal symmetric polyneuropathy	Yearly complete foot exam, visual foot exam each visit, daily exam by patient A1c, blood pressure, and lipid control	High risk of ulcers and charcot foot.	Management of glucose, lipids, and blood pressure Healthy BMI Medications: tricyclic antidepressants (amitriptyline, nortriptyline, imipramine), antiseizure drugs (gabapentin, carbamazepine,	Follow up with a podiatrist for recommendations and foot care Patient education regarding foot care, shoes, and signs and symptoms of problems See American Podiatric Medical

		pregabalin), serotonin and norepinephrine reuptake inhibitor (duloxetine), Substance P inhibitor (capsaicin cream)	Association at www.apma.org
Autonomic[‡] neuropathy: -Cardiac -Gastrointestinal -Sexual or bladder dysfunction -Sudomotor -Hypoglycemia unawareness -Pupillomotor	A1c, blood pressure, lipid control	Healthy BMI *Cardiac:* tachycardia—ACEI, beta-blockers Orthostatic hypotension—clonidine, midodrine, octreotide, mechanical measures *GI:* gastroparesis metoclopramide, erythromycin, small frequent meals, stay erect after meals for 1 hour *Sexual:* phosphodiesterase type 5 inhibitors, intracorporeal or intraurethral prostaglandins, vacuum devices, or penile prostheses *Bladder:* Bethanechol, intermittent self-catheterization *Sudomotor:* skin lubricants, vasodilators, scopolamine glycopyrrolate *Hypoglycemia:* set higher glucose goal, frequent glucose monitoring, continuous glucose monitor, insulin pump	Signs and symptoms: *Cardiac:* resting tachycardia, orthostatic hypotension, exercise intolerance *Gastrointestinal:* constipation, nausea, diarrhea, early fullness, erratic glucose levels, gastroparesis *Sexual or bladder:* erectile, bladder dysfunction, frequent UTIs *Sudomotor:* anhidrosis of the extremities, which may be accompanied by hyperhidrosis in the trunk[§] *Hypoglycemia:* inability to detect low glucose levels *Pupillomotor:* visual blurring, impaired adaption to ambient light

(continued)

Table 6.4 Prevention and Treatment of Diabetic Complications *(continued)*

	PREVENTION	PRECAUTIONS	TREATMENT*	COMMENTS
			Pupillomotor: care with night driving	
-Focal limb neuropathy -Proximal-motor neuropathy -Truncal radiculo-neuropathy	A1c, blood pressure, lipid control		*Focal limb:* surgery may be necessary *Proximal-motor neuropathy:* may require high-dose steroids or intravenous immunoglobulin *Truncal radiculo-neuropathy:* usually resolves in 4 to 6 months, treat with simple analgesics	*Focal limb:* entrapment syndromes such as carpel tunnel or trigger finger *Proximal-motor neuropathy:* occurs in older patients and presents with severe unilateral or bilateral muscle weakness and atrophy in the thighs *Truncal radiculo-neuropathy:* pain in the lower thoracic and abdominal wall unilaterally or bilaterally and is worse at night. Seen more frequently in older men
Dental disease	Daily brushing and flossing, regular dentist visits, healthy glucose levels		Healthy glucose control, dental visits every 6 months, smoking cessation, healthy lifestyle	Three times higher risk of severe periodontal disease if A1c >9, tooth loss, fungal infections, taste impairment, salivary gland dysfunction⁵
Sleep apnea	Healthy BMI Assessment each visit	Increased risk of heart disease, stroke, hypertension, and erectile dysfunction.	Weight loss, smoking cessation, avoid alcohol or sedatives at night, CPAP most effective, dental appliances	50% of patients with diabetes have sleep apnea⁸ Sleep lab study will confirm diagnosis
Coronary artery disease	Blood pressure, lipids, glucose, control, and	The major cause of morbidity and mortality.	In patients with known CVD, ACEI, statin, aspirin therapy should	CHF discontinue use of TZD Metformin may be used if patient

	healthy lifestyle and BMI Yearly assessment of risk factors, family history, presence of micro or macro-albuminuria		be used if no contraindications If MI, add a beta-blocker if not contraindicated Maintain lipid, glucose, and blood pressure control	has stable CHF and normal renal function Metformin should be discontinued if patient with CHF admitted to the hospital
Cerebrovascular disease (CVA)	Blood pressure, lipid, glucose control, and healthy lifestyle and BMI		Follow guidelines	80% of strokes are ischemic Occurs at a younger age in African Americans with HTN Smoking doubles the risk of CVA
Peripheral arterial disease (PAD)	Perform a screening ABI in patients >50 yr and diabetes for 10 yr or <50 yr if risk factors present Control blood pressure, lipids, and glucose, healthy lifestyle and BMI, smoking cessation	Higher risk of CVD, CVA, sudden death with PAD.	Walk indoors initially due to intermittent claudication and need to stop frequently, smoking cessation, antiplatelet medications (aspirin and clopidogrel)	Diagnostic ABI in any patient with symptoms of PAD—further vascular workup may be needed Many patients with PAD are asymptomatic

*From: American Diabetes Association. Standards of medical care in diabetes—2009. *Diabetes Care.* 2009;32:s13–s61.

†From: National Kidney Disease Education Program. Chronic kidney disease (CKD) information. Available at: http://www.nkdep.nih.gov/professionals/chronic_kidney_disease. htm#riskfactors. Accessed October 27, 2009.

‡From: American Association of Diabetes Educators. *The Art and Science of Diabetes Self-Management Education: A Desk Reference for Healthcare Professionals.* Chicago, Ill: American Association of Diabetes Educators; 2006:678.

§From: Vinik AI, Freeman R, Erbas T. Diabetic autonomic neuropathy: sudomotor dysfunction. Available at: http://www.medscape.com/viewarticle/473205_7. Accessed October 27, 2009.

¶From: American Dental Association. Diabetes and your oral health. Available at: http://www. ada.org/public/topics/diabetes_faq.asp#2. Accessed October 27, 2009.

#From: Medscape Nurses for the Web, Einhorn D, et al. Prevalence of sleep apnea in a population of adults with type 2 diabetes mellitus. Available at: http://www.medscape.com/ viewarticle/564208_4. Accessed October 27, 2009.

Diabetes Resource Toolkit

Patient Education

6–1 DIABETES CAN AFFECT ALL THESE PARTS OF YOUR BODY

Introduction

Diabetes affects the whole body. Here are some tips for good health with diabetes.

Eye

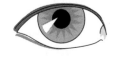

Recommendations:
1. See your doctor.
2. Control your blood glucose.
3. Control blood pressure.
4. Have your eyes checked yearly by an ophthalmologist (retinal eye exam).

Kidney

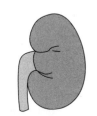

Recommendations:
1. Microalbumin test yearly.
2. See your doctor.
3. Control your blood glucose.
4. Control blood pressure.

Heart

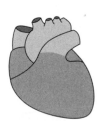

Recommendations:
1. See your doctor.
2. Control your blood glucose.
3. Follow a heart healthy diet low in saturated fat and cholesterol.
4. Control blood pressure.
5. Avoid smoking.
6. Exercise as directed.
7. Maintain a healthy weight.

Teeth and Gums

1. Brush gently with a soft toothbrush and floss after every meal.
2. Replace toothbrush every 3 months and after every cold and sore throat.
3. The best time to have dental work is when your blood glucose is in good control. Be sure to tell your dentist you have diabetes.

Sexual Health

- *Women*

  If you are thinking about having a baby, start working with your healthcare team before you get pregnant. In order to prevent complications, it is very important to have excellent control of your blood sugar levels when you conceive and throughout your pregnancy.

  Changes in hormonal levels during and before menstrual periods and menopause can affect your blood sugar levels. Check your blood sugar levels more frequently and talk to your healthcare team about making necessary changes to your care plan, if needed.

  High blood sugar levels may make you more prone to yeast infections.

  Diabetes can affect a woman's interest in sex due to depression or feeling tired from high blood sugar levels. Find someone on your healthcare team to talk with, and learn about medicines or counseling that can help.

- *Men*

  Impotence (erectile dysfunction, ED) may be related to diabetes or medications. Talk with your doctor or a urologist.

  Depression and lots of worry can lead to ED, and ED can cause men to feel depressed. Talk to your healthcare team if you have feelings of depression or too much worry. Medicine or counseling may help.

6–2 Foot Care for People with Diabetes

Help yourself prevent the complications of diabetes.
People with diabetes need to take special care of their feet.

1. Wash your feet daily with lukewarm water and soap.

2. Dry your feet well, especially between the toes.

3. Keep the skin supple with a moisturizing lotion (do not apply lotion between toes).

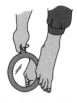

4. Check often for blisters, cuts, or sores. Tell your doctor if you find something wrong.

5. Use an emery board to shape toenails even with the ends of your toes.

6. Change daily into clean, soft socks or stockings, not too big or too small.

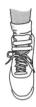

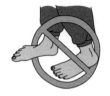

7. Keep your feet warm and dry. Preferably wear special padded socks and always wear shoes that fit well.

8. Never walk barefoot indoors or outdoors.

9. Examine your shoes every day for cracks, pebbles, nails, or anything that could hurt your feet.

Take good care of your feet—and use them! A brisk walk every day stimulates circulation.

6–3 DIABETES AND SLEEP

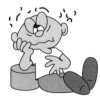

Getting the proper amount of sleep is essential to our well-being, especially for people with diabetes. When we don't get enough sleep, it can affect our health and our quality of life. Lack of proper sleep or disrupted sleep may result in:

- Weight Gain
- Increased Insulin Resistance
- Decreased Daytime Functioning

Sleep Disorders

Insomnia

- Do you have difficulty falling asleep?
- Do you have difficulty sleeping through the night?
- Do you still feel tired after waking up in the morning?

If you are experiencing the above symptoms, you may have a sleep disorder called insomnia. Please discuss this with your doctor as there are treatments to help deal with and/or prevent having insomnia.

Sleep Apnea

- Do you snore?
- Are you excessively tired during the day?
- Have you been told you stop breathing during sleep?
- Do you have a history of hypertension?
- Is your neck greater than 17 inches (male) or 16 inches (female) in circumference?

If you have 3 or more of the above symptoms, you may have a sleep disorder called *sleep apnea*. Sleep apnea is a serious disorder that involves obstruction of the upper airway. There are serious

Scripps Whittier
Diabetes Institute

consequences to your health associated with sleep apnea including hypertension, ischemic heart disease, stroke, driving-related accidents, and premature death. Please discuss this with your doctor as there are treatments for sleep apnea.

Restless Leg Syndrome

Do you have a "crawling" or "jittery" sensation that occurs in your legs and interferes with your ability to sleep?

This unpleasant sensation is called *restless leg syndrome,* which causes a strong urge to move the legs. This sensation can interfere with the ability to fall asleep or may even wake a person up from sleeping.

6–4 DIABETIC KETOACIDOSIS (DKA)

What is Ketoacidosis?

Ketoacidosis, or DKA, occurs when the body is not getting enough insulin. Acids called ketones travel through the blood, making you feel very sick by causing stomachache, nausea, and vomiting. DKA is more common in people with type 1 diabetes and is a major emergency. If this is not treated quickly, it may cause organ damage or even death.

What Can Cause Ketoacidosis?

1. Illness or infection
2. Missed taking your insulin or not getting enough insulin
3. Insulin that is no longer good or has expired
4. Insulin pump failure or insulin infusion set blockage
5. Blood sugar that is high, usually 200 or higher
6. A severe emotional or physical trauma

What are the Symptoms of Ketoacidosis?

1. Stomach pain, diarrhea (flu-like symptoms)
2. Nausea, vomiting
3. Generalized muscle pain, weakness
4. Fruity odor from breath
5. Rapid gasping breathing if not treated

When Should I Check for Urine Ketones?

1. Any time you have any of the symptoms or causes that are listed above

How Often Should I Check My Urine for Ketones?

1. Check your urine and your blood sugar every 4–5 hours

When Should I Call the Doctor?

1. If ketones are present, call your doctor immediately

6–5 MY HEALTH GOALS

My blood glucose goal for health, healing, and circulation: _____
My goal is to check my blood glucose at the following times:

_____ Breakfast _____ Lunch _____ Dinner _____ Bedtime

Healthy Glucose Goals

Lower Stress

Fun

Activity

Education

Medication

Healthy Food Choices

Choose One Goal for Healthy Blood Glucose:

Lower stress	Fun	Activity
Education	Medication	Food

How often? _____

The benefits to me: (circle answer or write in your own answer)
healthier A1c, feel better, better self-esteem, decrease stress

_____

_____

_____

_____

_____

Scripps Whittier
Diabetes Institute

©2009

References

1. National Kidney Disease Education Program. Chronic kidney disease (CKD) information. Available at: http://www.nkdep.nih.gov/professionals/chronic_kidney_disease.htm#riskfactors. Accessed October 27, 2009.

2. American Diabetes Association. Standards of medical care in diabetes—2010. *Diabetes Care.* 2010;33:S11–S61.

3. Bhavsar AR, Drouilhet JH. Retinopathy, diabetic, background. Available at: http://emedicine.medscape.com/article/1225122-overview. Accessed October 27, 2009.

4. American Association of Diabetes Educators. *The Art and Science of Diabetes Self-Management Education: A Desk Reference for Healthcare Professionals.* Chicago, IL: American Association of Diabetes Educators; 2006:678.

5. Vinik AI, Freeman R, Erbas T. Diabetic autonomic neuropathy: sudomotor dysfunction. Available at: http://www.medscape.com/viewarticle/473205_7. Accessed October 27, 2009.

6. Medscape Nurses for the Web, Einhorn D, et al. Prevalence of sleep apnea in a population of adults with type 2 diabetes mellitus. Available at: http://www.medscape.com/viewarticle/564208_4. Accessed October 27, 2009.

7. Babu AR, Herdegen J, Fogelfeld L, Shott S, Mazzone T. Type 2 diabetes, glycemic control, and continuous positive airway pressure in obstructive sleep apnea. *Arch Int Med.* February 28, 2005;165:447–452.

8. American Dental Association. Diabetes and your oral health. Available at: http://www.ada.org/public/topics/diabetes_faq.asp#2. Accessed October 27, 2009.

9. American Heart Association. PAD treatments and medications. Available at: http://www.americanheart.org/presenter.jhtml?identifier=3020257. Accessed October 27, 2009.

7 ▪ Blood Glucose Monitoring

Which Meter?

Blood glucose meters come in all shapes, sizes, colors; some are complex and have features to document activity, illness, pre- and post-glucose values, as well as insulin doses, all of which can be downloaded and printed into graphs or pie charts. And some are simple without a lot of extra features or memory storage. Almost every home blood glucose meter company has a meter that uses a test strip that wicks the blood from the finger, requires very little blood, and the meter no longer needs to be coded. These features increase the chance that the patient can successfully check his or her blood glucose appropriately and obtain a correct reading. The important issues related to blood glucose monitoring are that the patient comprehends how to use the glucose meter correctly, understands why he or she is checking the glucose at particular times, and knows what action to take related to the glucose results.

Depending on your state, insurance plans or health maintenance organizations may dictate which particular brand of meter is covered by the plan. Diabetes Health is a great online resource to view the latest blood glucose meters and their particular features; see www.diabeteshealth.com/charts. The January issue of *Diabetes Forecast* also lists home glucose meter information and can be located online at www.forecast.diabetes.org. **Table 7.1** lists several glucose meter manufacturers, their products, and their contact information.

Rationale for Home Blood Glucose Monitoring

- Safety
  - Prevent and detect hypoglycemia or hyperglycemia
  - Decrease the risk of diabetic ketoacidosis (DKA) with type 1 diabetes

- Medications
  - ○ Evaluate the effectiveness of oral or insulin mealtime therapies by checking a 2-hr postprandial glucose level
- Illness
  - ○ Monitor the effect of illness on the glucose level and treat accordingly
- Behavior change
  - ○ Directly see the effects of food, stress, and exercise on the glucose levels

Table 7.1 Home Blood Glucose Monitors

COMPANY AND METERS	TELEPHONE AND WEBSITE
Abbott Diabetes Care Freestyle, FreeStyle Lite, Precision Xtra (measures blood ketones)	888-522-5226 www.abbottdiabetescare.com
AgaMatrix Wave Sense Keynote	866-906-4197 www.wavesense.info
Bayer Contour, Breeze 2	800-348-8100 www.bayerdiabetes.com
Home Diagnostics True Track Smart System, SideKick, True Result	800-342-7226 www.homediagnosticsinc.com
LifeScan OneTouch Ultra, Ultra Smart, Ultra Mini, One Touch Ultra Link	800-227-8862 www.lifescan.com
Prodigy Prodigy Voice and Autocode, speaking meters	866-540-4786 www.prodigymeter.com
ReliOn NewTek, Ultima	888-922-0400 www.walmart.com
Roche Accu-Chek Advantage, Compact, Aviva, Compact Plus, Active	800-858-8072 www.accu-check.com

Blood Glucose Recommendations

The American Diabetes Association (ADA) makes the following recommendations for home blood glucose monitoring by patients.[1]

Type 2 Diabetes

- Set a regular schedule based on patient needs
- Consider the following times:
  - Alternate meals
  - Check before and 2 hours post meal
  - Bedtime to see if a snack is required
  - Before driving
  - Before and after exercise
  - Sick days
  - More often when adding or modifying therapy
- Pre meal: 70 mg/dL to 130 mg/dL
- Post meal: <180 mg/dL

Another rule of thumb for assessing the postmeal glucose and effectiveness of insulin or premeal orals is to have the patient check a premeal and a postmeal glucose. The postmeal glucose should be no more than 50 mg/dL higher than the premeal glucose.[2]

Type 1 Diabetes

- At least three times a day and usually more frequently for patients using multiple daily injections or an insulin pump
- Pre meal: 70 mg/dL to 130 mg/dL
- Post meal: <180 mg/dL

Another rule of thumb for assessing the postmeal glucose and effectiveness of insulin is to have the patient check a premeal and a postmeal glucose. The postmeal glucose should be no more than 50 mg/dL higher than the premeal glucose.[2]

Table 7.2 ADA Glucose Recommendations with Type I Diabetes		
	PREMEAL	BEDTIME
Toddlers/preschool up to age 6 yr	100–180 mg/dL	110–200 mg/dL
School age 6–12 yr	90–180 mg/dL	100–180 mg/dL
Adolescents and young adults 13–19 yr	90–130 mg/dL	90–150 mg/dL

Gestational Diabetes

- Fasting and 1 hr after a meal
- Goals: fasting less than 95 mg/dL; 1 hr after each main meal, 100 mg/dL to less than 140 mg/dL[3]

Blood Glucose Goals for Children and Young Adults[1]

Table 7.2 shows the ADA recommendations for blood glucose in children and adolescents with Type I diabetes.

Alternate Site Testing

Almost every new meter can be used for alternate site testing. The sites include forearm, palm of the hand, upper arm, or thigh. The concern, however, is that alternate site testing cannot accurately detect rapid blood glucose changes. For that reason, the Food and Drug Administration states alternate site testing is not to be used to evaluate hypoglycemia or hyperglycemia and should not be used by people who have hypoglycemia unawareness or women who are pregnant.[4] Alternate site testing may be used prior to a meal. The Food and Drug Administration does not recommend using alternate site testing after a meal, insulin dosing, or exercise unless more than 2 hours have passed from the onset of the meal, insulin dosing, or exercise. It is recommended to use the fingertips to check the glucose in those cases for accuracy.

Physician Role in Home Glucose Monitoring

- Provide the patient with a recommendation for frequency and timing of home blood glucose monitoring based on his or her current diabetes control, diabetes medications, and risk for hypoglycemia.
- Ask the patient to bring his or her home glucose records to your office at each visit or bring his or her personal meter, from which you can download the information. Many of the meter companies provide free software to download patient glucose results in your office.
- Spend a few minutes with the patient reviewing the glucose records together. This really does not take a lot of time and you are not only engaging the patient in his or her own self-care, but are validating the time the patient spends checking his or her blood sugar based on your recommendations. Both benefits are valuable and useful.

Insulin Pumps: Continuous Subcutaneous Insulin Infusion

One of the best ways to provide insulin therapy, the insulin pump continuously delivers insulin into the subcutaneous tissue, which allows for consistent insulin absorption which directly affects glucose levels. The vast majority of people using an insulin pump report a higher level of satisfaction related to flexibility with daily life and better glucose control. Although most often used by people with type 1 diabetes, those with type 2 diabetes on basal and bolus insulin can certainly use an insulin pump if they meet the criteria. Only rapid-acting insulin (lispro, aspart, glulisine) is used in the insulin pump.

The Medicare criteria for coverage of an insulin pump are as follows[5]:

- Fasting C-peptide level less than or equal to 110% of the lower limit of normal of the laboratory's measurement method
- The patient is taking at least three insulin injections a day

- History of recurring hypoglycemia
- Wide fluctuations in blood glucose before mealtime
- Dawn phenomenon with fasting glucose >200 mg/dL
- History of severe glycemic excursions
- The patient checks a blood glucose an average of at least four times a day (documented for 6 months prior to requesting an insulin pump)
- Continued coverage of the insulin pump would require the patient be seen and managed by a physician every 3 months

  Candidates for effective use of an insulin pump are as follows:

- Age: The patient can be any age. It is rare, but a patient may be as young as 6 months or in their 90s. Family members or other support persons may be involved in the management of the insulin pump if the person is unable to be independent with his or her care.
- Motivated and reliable: The patient is willing to check the blood glucose at least four times a day, keeps follow-up medical appointments, and uses the insulin pump per the manufacturer's guidelines.
- Diabetes type: Patients with type 1 or type 2 diabetes or those planning a pregnancy or pregnant and in need of better glucose control can use insulin pumps.
- Physically and mentally able: The patient must be able to comprehend the use of an insulin pump, respond appropriately to different situations related to using the pump, and has intact sensory and tactile functions to operate the pump safely.

How Does the Insulin Pump Work?

The Basal Component

The pump delivers a constant basal dose of insulin, which is programmed into the device. The starting time to set the basal dose for all insulin pumps is midnight. For example, the patient may set a basal rate from midnight to 4 a.m. of 0.6 unit per hour but increase the dose from 4 a.m. to 9 a.m. to 0.8 unit per hour if he or she tends to have higher glucose levels when waking up. From 9 a.m. to 6 p.m., the patient might require less insulin as a result of activity at work, and he or she may decrease the basal rate to 0.5 unit per hour. If the patient sits on the couch until bedtime, he or she might need to increase the dose to 0.6 unit per hour from 6 p.m. to midnight. The basal doses are very individualized based on the patient's glucose patterns. Most people require four to six different basal rates throughout the day.

Two methods to figure out the basal dose are as follows[2]:

- Reduce the prepump total daily dose (TDD) by 25% (reduce less if the prepump TDD is <70% rapid-acting insulin)
  - Example: The patient TDD is 50 units/day:
    $50 \times 0.75 = 38$ units/day (the new TDD, 50% to be used as basal insulin and 50% to be used as bolus insulin)
    $38 \div 2 = 19$ units basal dose
    19 units $\div$ 3 meals = 6 units for mealtime bolus
    19 units of basal $\div$ 24 hr = 0.8 units an hour as an initial starting basal dose
  - Basal doses would be revised based on the glucose patterns over 2 to 3 days.
- The second method is to take the patient's weight in kg and multiply it by 0.5 unit/day to get the total daily dose:
  - Example:
    82 kg $\times$ 0.5 = 41 TDD
    41 TDD $\div$ 2 = 21 units/day basal
    21 units $\div$ 3 meals = 7 units of bolus insulin at mealtime
    21 units of basal $\div$ 24 hr = 0.9 unit an hour as an initial starting dose
  - Basal doses would be revised based on the glucose patterns over 2 to 3 days.

The Bolus Component

The patient manually pushes a button on the insulin pump to deliver a bolus dose. A person's carbohydrate and correction ratio can be programmed into many of the insulin pumps so that the patient can enter the glucose level and amount of carbohydrate to be consumed, and then the insulin pump calculates how much insulin should be given based on those figures and in consideration of how much circulating insulin is still present from the last bolus dose. Even though the insulin pump calculates a certain dose, the patient must still decide whether that is the correct amount of insulin he or she wants to take based on his or her current status. For instance, is the patient going to take a walk after the meal or is he or she drinking alcohol with the meal? These factors may alter the amount of insulin the patient might take with the meal.

A method to figure out the mealtime bolus is as follows[2,6]:

- 500 ÷ TDD = Insulin to Carbohydrate ratio
- Example: 500 ÷ 38 = 13 grams of carbohydrate
- The person would bolus 1 unit of rapid-acting insulin for every 13 grams of carbohydrate consumed.

A method to figure out the correction bolus is this[2]:

- 1,700 ÷ TDD = Correction factor
- Example: 1,700 ÷ 38 = 45 mg/dL
- Therefore, 1 unit of rapid-acting insulin will drop the blood glucose by 45 points.

Here is an example of combining use of the carbohydrate and correction scales at a lunch meal. A person is to consume 60 g of carbohydrates for lunch, and premeal glucose is 225 mg/dL. The premeal glucose goal is 100 mg/dL. Total bolus dose for carbohydrates: 60 ÷ 13 = 4.6 units of bolus insulin (via insulin pump) to cover the mealtime carbohydrate. Then, 225 mg/dL (actual glucose) − 100 mg/dL (glucose goal) = 125 mg/dL ÷ 45 = 2.7 units to correct the glucose back to goal. Total insulin to be delivered is 4.6 + 2.7 = 7.3 units at lunch.

Benefits of the Pump

- Flexibility with mealtimes and snacks, timing and portions.
- Insulin delivery increments as low as 0.025 unit with some pumps.

- Ability to set temporary basal rates to assist in preventing exercise-related hypoglycemia both during and after exercise.
- Dual wave bolus (a combination of a regular bolus plus the square wave bolus) delivers a combination of immediate insulin bolus followed by an extended bolus (time to be determined by the patient). This is used to immediately address an elevated glucose and/or rapidly digesting carbohydrates in the meal plus provide additional insulin to cover high-fat foods such as pizza, which take longer to digest.
- Square wave bolus delivers a single dose of insulin over a time frame to be determined by the patient. This is used for a patient with gastroparesis to match insulin delivery to delayed gastric emptying or for the patient who is "grazing" (buffets, holiday parties) versus eating a single meal.

Precautions with an Insulin Pump
- The site and tubing should be changed every 3 days to prevent infection and clogging at the catheter insertion site.
- The sites should be rotated consistently to prevent lipohypertrophy. Poor insulin absorption may occur if the site is not rotated.
- Patients should remove the pump for any X-ray, CT scan, MRI, or radiation therapy and keep it out of the treatment area.[7]
- Patients should always change the infusion set, reservoir, and site during the day. They might not recognize if there is a problem with the system if they do this close to bedtime and then go to sleep.
- DKA can occur more often within 4 to 10 hr[8] with an insulin pump because of the short duration of the rapid-acting insulins. **Table 7.3** provides general guidelines on how to manage DKA while using an insulin pump.[2]

Insurance Coverage

Each insurance policy varies, and patients should call their agent to determine coverage benefits. Medicare patients pay 20% of the

Table 7.3   Diabetic Ketoacidosis

BLOOD GLUCOSE ≥250 MG/DL	KETONES PRESENT	KETONES NEGATIVE
Insulin Management	Inject a rapid-acting insulin via insulin syringe to verify administration.	Give a correction bolus via the insulin pump. Recheck glucose in 1 hr. If glucose is not lower, give injection with an insulin syringe.
Pump Management	Change the pump infusion set and insulin and reinsert the catheter in a new location.	Change the pump infusion set and insulin and reinsert the catheter in a new location.
Follow-Up	Monitor glucose every 1 to 2 hr. If glucose levels are not improving, call your healthcare provider. If nausea, vomiting, diarrhea, or change in physical status occurs, go to the Emergency Room immediately. Call 911.	Continue to monitor glucose levels and ketones. Call your healthcare provider if your glucose levels are not improving within several hours.

Medicare-approved amount after the yearly Part B deductible. Medicare then pays 80% of the cost of the insulin pump. Medicare also pays for the insulin that is used with the insulin pump.

For more information about durable medical equipment and diabetes supplies, patients can call 1-800-633-4227 and see www.medicare.gov/Publications/Pubs/pdf/11022.pdf. **Table 7.4** lists insulin pump resources. Also, Diabetes Health features insulin pump information at www.diabeteshealth.com/charts. And, as mentioned earlier, the January issue of *Diabetes Forecast* also lists insulin pump information and can be located online at www.forecast.diabetes.org.

Table 7.4   Insulin Pump Resources

Animas Corporation, Animas One Touch Ping System: www.animascorp.com, 877-937-7867

Medtronic, Minimed Paradigm Pumps: www.minimed.com, 866-948-6633

Insulet Corporation, Omnipod Pump: www.myomnipod.com, 800-591-3455

Disetronic Medical Systems, Accu-Check Spirit Pump: www.disetronic-usa.com, 800-280-7801

Sooil Development, Dana IIS Pump: www.sooil.com, 866-747-6645

Insulin Pumper Group: www.insulin-pumpers.org

Children with Diabetes: www.childrenwithdiabetes.com

NIPRO Diabetes Systems, Amigo insulin pump: www.NIPRODIABETES.com, 888-651-7867

Continuous Glucose Monitoring

Similar to inserting an insulin pump, the continuous glucose sensor is inserted into the subcutaneous tissue and measures glucose from interstitial fluid. The sensor can be left in place for 72 hours to a week (depending on the manufacturer). The continuous glucose monitoring (CGM) device has two components: a sensor, which includes the transmitter, and a receiver, which receives glucose data from the sensor. The Minimed Paradigm insulin pump has a receiver built into the insulin pump. The DexCom Seven, the Abbott Freestyle Navigator, and the Guardian Real Time System all have a handheld receiver.

Who Is a Candidate for CGM?

- Both the DexCom Seven and the Abbott Freestyle Navigator are approved for adults 18 years and older. The Minimed Paradigm Real Time System and the Guardian Real Time System are approved for children age 7 and older and adults.[9]
- The continuous glucose monitor can be used with type 1 or type 2 diabetes.

- A small study done in Europe and reported in the *British Medical Journal* found that pregnant women who had diabetes and who were placed on CGM had 64% lower risk of macrosomia and 0.6% lower absolute glycosylated hemoglobin levels compared to standard care. Further studies should be done to validate the results.[9]

Benefits of CGM

- Alarm system vibrates or gives an audible response to a low or high glucose level, which is programmed in by the patient based on individual-specific limits.
- Trend arrows alarm if a rapid drop or rise in glucose is detected.
- Glucose results are displayed every 5 minutes on the receiver for the DexCom Seven and Minimed Paradigm. The Abbott Freestyle Navigator displays every 1 minute.
- Flexibility—some people use the CGM device when there is a change in their blood glucose patterns and they want to see what the 24-hr glucose pattern is so that they can change basal or bolus rates on their insulin pump.
- CGM can provide peace of mind for people with hypoglycemia unawareness or nocturnal hypoglycemia.
- Software is available to download glucose results onto a computer.
- Studies have shown a reduction in A1c by 0.5% in adults age 25 and older who make appropriate insulin or lifestyle changes based on the CGM data.[1]

Precautions with CGM

- Setup (2 to 10 hr) and a calibration time (12 to 72 hr) are required for all devices, which involves self blood glucose monitoring.
- CGM does not replace self blood glucose monitoring. It is recommended that patients check the blood glucose with

a meter to verify hypoglycemia or hyperglycemia results before making any treatment decisions.

- There is a 10- to 15-minute lag time between the interstitial glucose reading and blood glucose reading.
- The receiver must be within 5 to 10 feet of the sensor to transmit glucose levels.

Insurance Coverage

- More insurance companies are now including CGM as a benefit.
- A letter of necessity might be required by the insurance company.
- Out-of-pocket cost may range from $800 to $1,339 for the monitor and $35 to $60 for the sensors.[10]

Table 7.5 lists resources related to CGM.

Table 7.5 Resources for CGM
Medtronic, Guardian Real Time System and the Paradigm Real Time System: www.minimed.com, 866-948-6633
Abbott Diabetes Care, Freestyle Navigator: www.contiuousmonitor.com, 866-597-5520
DexCom, DexCom Seven: www.dexcom.com, 877-633-9266

Diabetes Resource Toolkit

Patient Education

7–1 How Often Should I Test My Blood Glucose?

7–2 Suggested Goals for Blood Glucose

7–1 How Often Should I Test My Blood Glucose?

Your doctor and diabetes team will tell you how often you should test your blood glucose. Testing frequency may vary for many reasons.

If you have type 1 diabetes, you will most likely be asked to check 3 to 4 times a day. If you have newly diagnosed type 2 diabetes, you may be asked to check 1 to 3 times a day, depending on your medication. People with type 2 diabetes who have stable blood glucose levels may need to check only 1 or 2 times a week. Do check your blood glucose anytime you do not feel right to make sure your blood sugar is in a safe range.

In order to get a true picture of the entire day, it is important that you vary the times of day that you test. The fasting blood glucose (before you eat) usually varies the least and reflects the output of sugar by the liver in the early morning hours. The peak blood glucose level after meals is generally reached 1 to 2 hours following the meal. Because of this, testing after a meal will give you the most information about how high your blood glucose rises. If your carbohydrate intake was too high, you will see a higher blood glucose level reflected in your 2-hour, postmeal blood glucose check.

I will test my blood glucose at the following times: place a check mark:

TIME	SUNDAY	MONDAY	TUESDAY	WEDNESDAY	THURSDAY	FRIDAY	SATURDAY
Before breakfast							
2 hours after breakfast							
Before lunch							
2 hours after lunch							
Before evening meal							
2 hours after evening meal							
Bedtime							

7–2 SUGGESTED GOALS FOR BLOOD GLUCOSE

	IDEAL	ACTION SUGGESTED
Fasting and Pre Meal	70–130 mg/dL	Over 140 mg/dL
2-hr Post Meal	<180 mg/dL	Over 180 mg/dL
Bedtime	100–140 mg/dL	Less than 100 mg/dL

Your individual goal may vary.

Scripps Whittier
Diabetes Institute

References

1. American Diabetes Association. Standards of medical care in diabetes—2009. *Diabetes Care.* 2009;32:s13–s61.

2. Bode B. *Pumping Protocol: A Physician Guide to Insulin Pumping Therapy Initiation.* 2008:13. Supported by an educational grant from MiniMed.

3. American Diabetes Association. 2009 ADA Standards of Care. *Diabetes Care.* 2009;32:s-22.

4. US Food and Drug Administration. Medical devices: glucose testing devices. Available at: http://www.fda.gov/MedicalDevices/Products andMedicalProcedures/InVitroDiagnostics/GlucoseTestingDevices/ default.htm. Accessed October 28, 2009.

5. US Department of Health and Human Services, Centers for Medicare and Medicaid Services. *Coverage Issues Manual.* Baltimore, Md: Centers for Medicare and Medicaid Services; September 26, 2001. Available at: http://cms.hhs.gov/transmittals/downloads/R143CIM .pdf. Accessed October 28, 2009.

6. Walsh J, Roberts R. *Pumping Insulin.* 4th ed. San Diego, CA: Torrey Pines Press; 2006.

7. Medtronic. Diabetes management. Available at: http://www. medtronic.com/our-therapies/diabetes-management/index.htm. Accessed October 28, 2009.

8. Diabetes Health. Product reference guide: Dec. 2008/Jan. 2009. Available at: http://www.diabeteshealth.com/charts/. Accessed October 28, 2009.

9. Barclay L, Vega C. Continuous glucose monitoring during pregnancy may improve outcomes. MedscapeCME. Available at: http://cme. medscape.com/viewarticle/581108?src=rss. Accessed October 28, 2009.

10. Diabetes Mall. Comparison of current continuous monitors. Available at: http://www.diabetesnet.com/diabetes_technology/continuous_ monitoring.php. Accessed October 28, 2009.

8 ▪ Diabetes and Cultural Considerations

Minorities, underserved, and underinsured populations are at high risk for diabetes and have less access to timely diabetes care than do non-minorities and those with insurance. Few diabetes management and education programs have been adapted or shown to be effective for these populations. Among those with diabetes, Mexican Americans and African Americans are less likely to be insured or have access to traditional primary care and preventive health care.

Healthcare providers in safety net settings are the primary providers of care to the majority of low-income and ethnic populations with diabetes. In California, community clinics and health centers make up the fabric of the safety net and provide care to nearly 4 million patients annually, two thirds of whom live below the poverty line. These healthcare providers are frequently in rural areas without access to ongoing professional education; or they are in busy and underfunded clinics that cannot afford to send them away for extensive professional training. This situation is not uncommon in many other parts of the United States.

California alone has more than 2 million people with diabetes. By the year 2020, the prevalence of diabetes in California is expected to exceed 4 million people. Ethnically diverse populations are disproportionately affected by diabetes. African Americans are 1.4 to 2.2 times more likely than Caucasians to have diabetes; the comparable figure for American Indians is 2.8. In addition, Hispanic Americans are more likely to have diabetes than are non-Hispanics, whereas Japanese Americans, Chinese Americans, Filipino Americans, and Korean Americans are also at increased risk.[1–4]

Project Dulce, a program of Scripps Whittier Diabetes Institute, has 10 years of experience implementing diabetes care and self-management education programs based on a chronic care model and multidisciplinary team approach. Project Dulce shares this expertise with safety net providers and community health centers by providing group and individual training and technical assistance to help them build their capacity to manage chronic diseases.[5,6]

Project Dulce's Program Design

The goals of Project Dulce are to improve the health of under-served, ethnically diverse persons with diabetes by integrating nurse-led management and peer education in their primary care home. The model was designed in 1996–1997 by a broad collaboration of health agencies and providers in San Diego County to address the problem of poorly controlled diabetes among un- and underinsured persons, specifically Latinos but later broadened to Vietnamese, Filipinos, and African Americans. This collaboration brought together experts in state-of-the-art diabetes care with those experienced in providing services to low-income, ethnically diverse populations. The result was a model that linked clinical excellence with cultural relevance.

Project Dulce is designed to be implemented in community health center settings. Project Dulce has since been adapted to operate effectively in the university health system and private practice settings. The program has provided care to more than 8,000 patients and currently maintains an active patient population of 2,500 in its electronic registry.

Use of Multidisciplinary Care Teams

Project Dulce's multidisciplinary care teams consist of a nurse manager (registered nurse [RN]/Certified Diabetes Educator [CDE]), dietitian, medical assistant (MA), and peer educator. The goals of the team are to meet the American Diabetes Association (ADA) standards of care and to achieve improvements in HbA1c, blood pressure, and lipid parameters and health behaviors. The

RN/CDEs have extensive experience in diabetes education and are further trained to use the protocols in Staged Diabetes Management (SDM) for glucose, lipid, and hypertension management.[7] Each participant receives a 1-hr baseline visit to assess demographic information, a diabetes history, weight, blood pressure, foot exam (including neurosensory and vascular exam), HbA1c, chemistry and lipid panel, liver function tests, and proteinuria. Diabetes mellitus (DM) self-management guidelines and goals are reviewed in the initial patient visit. The RN/CDEs provide recommendations for changes in diabetes medications, following SDM protocols, to the primary care provider (PCP), with whom they work closely to ensure consensus with the recommended treatment plan. The prescriptions are written by the PCP. The RN/CDE is responsible for ordering follow-up labs and scheduling return visits. If there are multiple diabetes issues to manage, a follow-up visit is usually scheduled within the next 2 weeks. The patients are seen a minimum of four times per year. Blood pressure, weight, and HbA1c values are obtained at each quarterly visit and additional labs as dictated by the SDM protocols. Self-monitored blood glucose results are reviewed at each visit.

The MA is responsible for translation (primarily Spanish to English), taking vitals, phlebotomy, and patient reminders. Bilingual-bicultural dietitians deliver general dietary information and specific carbohydrate counting education depending on the patient's needs. Most patients receive two 45-minute dietary visits per year.

Peer-Led Diabetes Self-Management Education

Project Dulce has built upon the effectiveness of community health workers in mediating cultural barriers to care and education by providing extensive training to enable them to be effective diabetes peer educators. Persons with diabetes that exemplify the traits of a "natural leader" are identified from the patient population and recruited to be trained. The Project Dulce peer education program comprises a 4-month, competency-based training and mentoring program. Each potential peer educator is required to complete a series of diabetes classes as a patient, and then to co-teach the series with an experienced health educator. Each peer educator must successfully master the competencies required in each training phase before proceeding to the subsequent phase of training, and finally graduating as a diabetes peer educator.

Referrals to classes are made by the nurse manager at the patient's initial visit and are supported by the patient's PCP. Peer educators also make follow-up calls to encourage class attendance. Classes are held at times convenient to patients at each clinic site, including evenings.

The diabetes education curriculum delivered by the peers (*promotoras*) consists of eight 2-hr sessions (one per week). It is very graphic and has been adapted for use in Latino, African American, Filipino, and Vietnamese populations through extensive cultural research and testing. **Figure 8.1** shows a sample of chapters of the curriculum. **Figure 8.2** shows a Spanish language handout demonstrating healthy actions to manage diabetes. **Figure 8.3**

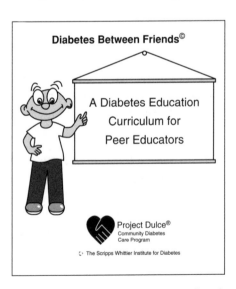

■ **Figure 8.1** **Scripps Whittier Project Dulce, "Diabetes Between Friends" Curriculum Cover**

shows an English language handout showing visual and written signs and symptoms of hypoglycemia.

Classes are taught in patients' and *promotoras*' native language and cover DM and its complications; the role of diet, exercise, and medication; and the importance of self-monitoring of glucose levels. Each class includes interactive sessions, providing opportunities for patients to discuss their personal experiences and beliefs about diabetes. The groups are interactive, and each group member provides support and advice to other members of the group. Peer educators present factual information about diabetes and its management and address cultural beliefs and myths that may interfere with optimum management, such as the fear of using insulin or the reliance on urine or nopales (prickly pear

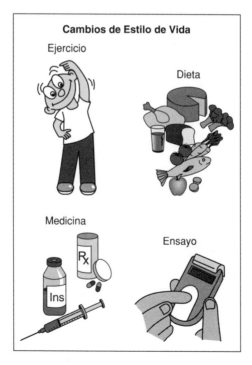

■ **Figure 8.2** **Scripps Whittier Project Dulce Spanish language handout demonstrating healthy actions to manage diabetes**

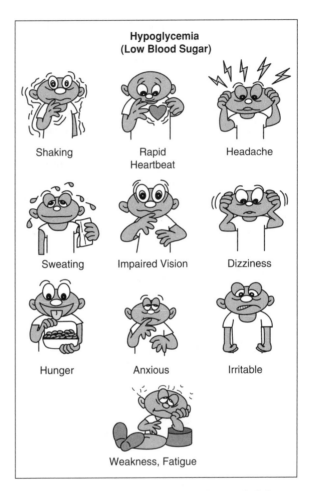

■ Figure 8.3 **Scripps Whittier Project Dulce English language handout showing visual and written signs and symptoms of hypoglycemia**

cactus) in an attempt to cure DM. Cooking, exercise, and stress reduction demonstrations enhance the information presented. Exchange of personal stories and fears about DM is encouraged and is meant to enable the patients to bond with each other and discuss their fears. Graduation ceremonies, which include family members, celebrate the successful completion of the course, and graduates are encouraged to continue to be involved in monthly support groups.

All the elements of ADA-recognized teaching programs are covered during the course of the classes. Peer educators are familiar with the community healthcare clinic system and encourage the patients to return for visits with their providers for more information about their diabetes management.

Project oversight is provided by a board-certified endocrinologist acting as medical director of Project Dulce. Medical questions encountered by the RN/CDE team are first taken to the PCP within the community clinic, and unresolved issues or difficult decisions are made in consultation with the endocrinologist. Medical education forums are conducted twice a year to update PCPs and their staff on the latest approaches to diabetes care. An operations manager meets regularly with each site's implementation team to problem-solve any logistical or procedural issues. A community-based steering committee composed of community health leaders, clinic providers, Project Dulce team members, and program participants review the progress of the program on a regular basis.

Multilingual patient education handouts have been developed and are available for download at the Scripps Whittier Diabetes Institute website (www.whittier.org). Samples are attached in the Diabetes Resource Toolkit at the end of this chapter (as well as on the CD-ROM). The training curriculum for community health workers is available through the training center of Scripps Whittier Diabetes Institute.

Examples of Cultural Considerations in Diets

Latino Culture

The usual diet is high in salt, sugar, starches, and fats. The Hispanic and Latino cultures ascribe to the *hot* and *cold* food theories. Many illnesses are believed to be caused by a disruption of the hot and cold balances in the body. Eating foods of the opposite variety may cure or prevent specific hot and cold diseases.

Food is considered a celebration, as it is for many other cultures. Many family gatherings center around food. Staples include rice, beans, and flour and corn tortillas. Tortillas treated with calcium carbonate provide much-needed calcium in the Mexican American diet.

Traditional Mexican American and other Hispanic/Latin mealtimes vary from those in the United States. The main meal of the day is usually eaten between 2 and 3 p.m., and the evening meal is generally served between 9 and 9:30 p.m. The healthcare provider must be aware of these time differences to adjust medications and other therapies as needed.

African American Culture

Traditionally prepared soul food is often high in fat, sodium, and starch. Highly suited to the physically demanding lives of laborers and farmhands and rural lifestyles in general, it is now a contributing factor to obesity, heart disease, and diabetes in a population that has become increasingly more urban and sedentary.

As a result, more health-conscious African Americans are using alternative methods of preparation, eschewing trans fats in favor of natural vegetable oils and substituting smoked turkey for fatback and other cured pork products; limiting the amount of refined sugar in desserts; and emphasizing the consumption of more fruits and vegetables than animal protein. There is some resistance to such changes, however, because they involve deviating from long-held culinary tradition.

Native American Culture

As with many other cultures, food has more of a meaning than just nutrition. Food is the focal point of many family and religious celebrations. Women may work several days preparing large amounts of food for important events.

Diet consists of various meats and chicken. The Navajo people often eat sheep as a main source of meat. Lard is used for cooking. Gallbladder disease is somewhat common among Native Americans because of high-fat diets. Diet-induced gallbladder disease has been documented in children as young as 11 years of age.

Herbs are used in the treatment of many illnesses to cleanse the body of poisons and ill spirits. Upon treatment, it is important for the healthcare provider to consider the herbs that the patient may be taking to avoid herbal interactions with certain medications.

Lactose intolerance is common in Native Americans. Vitamin D deficiency occurs frequently because of decreased milk intake. Some tribal rites require food restrictions and can produce episodes of malnutrition, especially in children.

Asian Cultures

The dietary preferences described for the various Asian cultures are often traditional preferences. Asian people who have lived in the United States for years may change their dietary preferences as they acculturate to American ways. Healthcare providers must investigate preferences on an individual basis to avoid stereotyping in any manner.

For many Asian people, food is more than nourishment. It is often a fundamental form of socialization: they may actually bring more food to work than necessary in order to share the food with coworkers.

- Steamed or fried rice is eaten at almost every meal and is served with fish, meat, pork, and vegetables.
- There is a high incidence of lactose intolerance among adults of some Asian cultures.

Polynesian Culture

Coconut cream may be used in the preparation of food, which tends to be high in calories. Historically, Polynesian people have valued a larger, heavier body. Obesity has led to diabetes, heart attacks, and strokes and is the main cause of death in this group of people. Exercising and dieting are beginning to be encouraged.

Diabetes Resource Toolkit
Patient Education

English

8–1 ABCs of Diabetes Management

8–2 Blood Sugar Levels and Target Numbers

8–3 Foot Care for People with Diabetes

8–4 Treatments Used in Diabetes

Spanish

8–5 ABCs of Diabetes Management

8–6 Blood Sugar Levels and Target Numbers

8–7 How to Read a Food Label

8–8 Treatments Used in Diabetes

Chinese

8–9 ABCs of Diabetes Management

8–10 Blood Sugar Levels and Target Numbers

8–11 How to Read a Food Label

Vietnamese

8–12 ABCs of Diabetes Management

8–13 Blood Sugar Levels and Target Numbers

8–14 How to Read a Food Label

8–1 ABCs of Diabetes Management

Testing for A1c, Blood Pressure, and Cholesterol

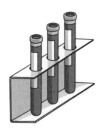

A1c = Glycosylated Hemoglobin, Glycohemoglobin (blood test) can report a blood sugar level average over a period of 2–3 months. The American Diabetes Association's recommended level for A1c is below 7%.

Blood Pressure

The top numbers (systolic) and bottom numbers (diastolic) tell you the force of the blood inside your artery walls. The American Diabetes Association's recommended level for blood pressure is below 130/80 mm Hg.

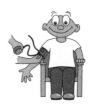

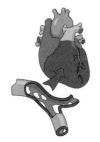

Cholesterol = Lipid Panel, Lipoprotein (blood test)

The American Diabetes Association's recommended level for total cholesterol is below 200 mg/dL, LDL below 100 mg/dL, HDL above 40 mg/dL in men and above 50 mg/dL in women, and triglycerides below 150 mg/dL.

PROJECT DULCE™
DIABETES EXCELLENCE ACROSS COMMUNITIES

8–2 BLOOD SUGAR LEVELS AND TARGET NUMBERS

Pre-Diabetes	100–125 mg/dL
	A1c 5.7 to 6.4%
Diagnosis of Diabetes	126 mg/dL or above fasting on two separate tests
	or
	200 mg/dL or above on random test with the presence of symptoms of diabetes
	or
	A1c ≥ 6.5%

Target Levels*

Fasting	70–130 mg/dL
2 hr after the first bite of a meal	Below 180 mg/dL
At bedtime	100–140 mg/dL
Hypoglycemia (low blood sugar)	Below 70 mg/dL
Hyperglycemia (high blood sugar)	Above 180 mg/dL

Note: Based on the American Diabetes Association's Clinical Practice Recommendations 2010. Your diabetes team may individualize these target numbers.

Scripps Whittier
Diabetes Institute

8–3 FOOT CARE FOR PEOPLE WITH DIABETES

People with diabetes need to take special care of their feet.

1. Wash your feet daily with lukewarm water and soap.

2. Dry your feet well, especially between the toes.

3. Keep the skin supple with a moisturizing lotion (do not apply lotion between toes).

4. Check often for blisters, cuts, or sores. Tell your doctor if you find something wrong.

5. Use an emery board to shape toenails even with the ends of your toes.

6. Change daily into clean, soft socks or stockings. Make sure you wear the correct size.

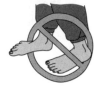

7. Keep your feet warm and dry. Always wear shoes that fit well and, if possible, wear special padded socks.

8. Never go barefoot— inside or outdoors.

9. Examine your shoes every day for damage or debris (pebbles, nails, etc.) that could injure your feet.

Take good care of your feet—and use them!
A brisk walk every day stimulates circulation.

Foot Care for People with Diabetes
Translation of this publication was supported by HRSA HCAP Grant # G92OA02204.
©2009 The Whittier Institute for Diabetes

Permission granted by The Whittier Institute for Diabetes to copy for patient education purposes. For additional information see www.whittier.org

PROJECT DULCE™
DIABETES EXCELLENCE ACROSS COMMUNITIES

PROJECT DULCE™
DIABETES EXCELLENCE ACROSS COMMUNITIES

8–4 TREATMENTS USED IN DIABETES

Action sites of diabetes medications:

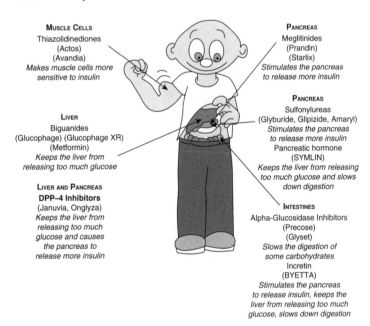

MUSCLE CELLS
Thiazolidinediones
(Actos)
(Avandia)
*Makes muscle cells more
sensitive to insulin*

PANCREAS
Meglitinides
(Prandin)
(Starlix)
*Stimulates the pancreas
to release more insulin*

PANCREAS
Sulfonylureas
(Glyburide, Glipizide, Amaryl)
*Stimulates the pancreas
to release more insulin*
Pancreatic hormone
(SYMLIN)
*Keeps the liver from releasing
too much glucose and slows
down digestion*

LIVER
Biguanides
(Glucophage) (Glucophage XR)
(Metformin)
*Keeps the liver from
releasing too much glucose*

LIVER AND PANCREAS
DPP–4 Inhibitors
(Januvia, Onglyza)
*Keeps the liver from
releasing too much
glucose and causes
the pancreas to
release more insulin*

INTESTINES
Alpha-Glucosidase Inhibitors
(Precose)
(Glyset)
*Slows the digestion of
some carbohydrates*
Incretin
(BYETTA)
*Stimulates the pancreas
to release insulin, keeps the
liver from releasing too much
glucose, slows down digestion*

8–5 LO BÁSICO EN EL CUIDADO DE LA DIABETES

Pruebas para A1c, Presión Arterial y Colesterol

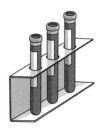

A1c = Hemoglobina Glicosilada, Glicohemoglobina (prueba de sangre) puede indicar el nivel promedio de glucosa en la sangre durante un periodo de 2 a 3 meses.

El nivel de A1c recomendado por la Asociación Americana de la Diabetes es menor al 7%.

Presión Arterial

Numero superior (presión sistólica) y numero inferior (presión diastólica) indican la fuerza de la sangre dentro de las arterias. El nivel de presión arterial recomendado por la Asociación Americana de la Diabetes es menor a 130/80 mm/Hg.

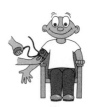

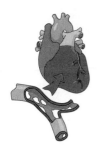

Colesterol = Perfil de lípidos, Lipoproteína (prueba de sangre). El nivel de colesterol total que recomienda la Asociación Americana para la Diabetes sea menor a 200 mg/dl, LDL (Lípidos de Baja Densidad) menor a 100 mg/dl, HDL (Lípidos de Alta Densidad) mayor a 40 mg/dl en los hombres y mayor a 50 mg/dl en las mujeres, y triglicéridos menor a 150 mg/dl.

8-6 Niveles de Glucosa en la Sangre y Números Meta

Pre-Diabetes	100–125 mg/dL
	A1c 5.7 to 6.4%
Diagnóstico de Diabetes	126 mg/dl en ayunas en dos pruebas separadas
	O
	200 mg/dl o mayor en pruebas aleatorias con la presencia de síntomas de diabetes
	O
	A1c ≥ 6.5%

Niveles Meta*

En ayunas	70–130 mg/dL
2 horas después de los alimentos	Menor de 180 mg/dL
A la hora de acostarse	100–140 mg/dL
Hipoglucemia (glucosa baja en las sangre)	Menor de 70 mg/dL
Hiperglucemia (glucosa alta en la sangre)	Mayor de 180 mg/dL

*Según las Recomendaciones del 2010 de Práctica Clínica de la Asociación Americana para la Diabetes. Su equipo contra la diabetes puede individualizar estos números meta

Scripps Whittier
Diabetes Institute

8–7 ¡LEA LA ETIQUETA DE VALOR NUTRICIONAL!

Tamaño de las Porciones. Los datos nutricionales que aparecen en la etiqueta son "por porción". Todas las cifras mencionadas en la etiqueta son las cantidades en una porción. Si va a comer más de una porción, necesita ajustar las cifras de acuerdo a esto. Por ejemplo, si el tamaño de la porción es de 1 taza y usted va a comer 2 tazas, necesita duplicar todas las cifras mencionadas en la etiqueta nutricional.

PRODUCTO – YOGUR SIN SABOR

Total de Grasa/Colesterol- Para seguir una dieta baja en grasa, elija botanas, cereales, productors lácteos, platillos de acompañamiento y carnes bajas en grasa que contengan 3 gramos o menos de grasa por porción. Las carnes y los quesos deben de tener 5 gramos o menos de grasa por porción.

Grasas saturadas o trans –Las grasas saturadas o trans pueden causar que su nivel de colesterol se eleve. Elija alimentos con menos de 1/3 de grasa en grasas saturadas y cero grasas trans.

Valor Nutricional

Tamaño de Porción 1 Taza (248 g)
Porciones por Paquete 4

Cantidad por Porción

Calorías 150   Calorías de Grasa 35

	% del Valor Díario*
Grasa Total 4 g	**6%**
Grasa Saturada 2.5 g	**12%**
Grasa Trans 0 g	
Colesterol 20 mg	**7%**
Sodio 170 mg	**7%**
Total de Carbohidratos 17 g	**6%**
Fibra Dietética 0 g	**0%**
Azúcar 17 g	
Proteina 13 g	

Vitamina A 4%	•	Vitamina C 6%
Calcío 40%	•	Hierro 0%

*El valor de porcentaje diario está basado en una dieta de 2,000 calorías. Su valor diario puede ser mayor 0 menor dependiendo en la necesidad de sus calorias:

		Calorias:	2,000	2,500
Grasa Total	Menos de		65 g	80 g
Grasa Saturada	Menos de		20 g	25 g
Colesterol	Menos de		300 mg	300 mg
Sodio	Menos de		2,400 mg	2,400 mg
Total de Carbohidratos			300 g	375 g
Fibra Dietetica			25 g	30 g

Calorías por gramo:
Grasa 9 • Carbohidrato 4 • Proteina 4

Sodio –Para seguir una dieta baja en sodio, elija alimentos que contengan el 5% o menos del valor diario de sodio. Los alimentos que contienen el 20% o más son considerados alimentos con alto contenido de sodio.

Total de Carbohidratos –Esta es la cantidad en gramos que usted debe de usar para determinar a cuántas porciones de carbohidratos equivale este alimento. Una porción de carbohidratos equivale a 15 gramos de carbohidratos totales.

Fibra –Trate de consumer de 25 a 35 gramos de fibra diariamente. Si hay 5 o más gramos de fibra, estos pueden restarse de los gramos de carbohidratos cuando se calculen las porciones de carbohidratos.

Azúcares –La cantidad de gramos de azúcar ya está calculada como parte de los carbohidratos totales. No use esta cifra para calcular las porciones de carbohidratos.

Vitaminas y minerales –Su meta es del 100% de cada una diariamente. Comer una variedad de alimentos diariamente le ayudará a alcanzar esta meta.

8–8 TRATAMIENTOS UTILIZADOS EN EL MANEJO DE LA DIABETES

Los medicamentos para la diabetes son pastillas que bajan el nivel de glucosa en la sangre.

Estas pastillas *no* son insulina.

Sitios donde actúan los medicamentos para la diabetes:

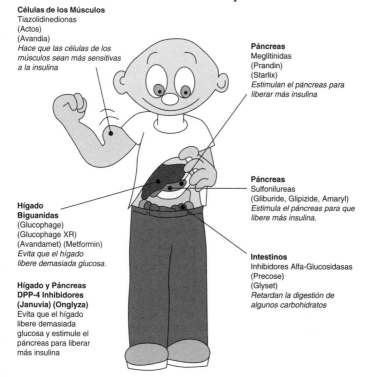

Células de los Músculos
Tiazolidinedionas
(Actos)
(Avandia)
Hace que las células de los músculos sean más sensitivas a la insulina

Páncreas
Meglitinidas
(Prandin)
(Starlix)
Estimulan el páncreas para liberar más insulina

Páncreas
Sulfonilureas
(Gliburide, Glipizide, Amaryl)
Estimula el páncreas para que libere más insulina.

Hígado
Biguanidas
(Glucophage)
(Glucophage XR)
(Avandamet) (Metformin)
Evita que el hígado libere demasiada glucosa.

Intestinos
Inhibidores Alfa-Glucosidasas
(Precose)
(Glyset)
Retardan la digestión de algunos carbohidratos

Hígado y Páncreas
DPP-4 Inhibidores
(Januvia) (Onglyza)
Evita que el hígado libere demasiada glucosa y estimule el páncreas para liberar más insulina

8–9 糖尿病管理入門
檢驗 A1c、血壓及膽固醇

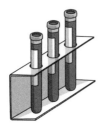

A1c = 糖化血色素，Glycohemoglobin (驗血)可以報告 2-3 個月當中血糖含量平均值。美國糖尿病協會推薦 A1c 標準低於 7%。

血壓

高壓(收縮)與低壓(舒張)可以看出動脈壁內血液的力量。美國糖尿病協會推薦血壓標準低於 130/80 mm/Hg。

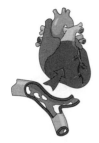

膽固醇 = 脂質檢驗，脂蛋白 (驗血)

美國糖尿病協會建議膽固醇標準低於 200 mg/dl，LDL (低密度脂蛋白)低於 100 mg/dl，HDL (高密度脂蛋白) 男性高於 40 mg/dl，女性高於 50 mg/dl，三酸甘油脂低於 150 mg/dl。

Chinese - ABC's of Diabetes Management
Translation of this publication was supported by HRSA HCAP Grant # G92OA02204.
©2009 The Whittier Institute for Diabetes

PROJECT DULCE™
DIABETES EXCELLENCE ACROSS COMMUNITIES

8–10 血糖含量及指標

前糖尿病期   100–125 mg/dL
A1c 5.7–6.4%

糖尿病診斷   126 mg/dL 或高於
禁食後分兩次檢測

或

200 mg/dL 或高於
糖尿病症狀時抽檢

或

A1c ≥6.5%

目標程度

禁食   70–130 mg/dL

進第一口食物後兩小時   低於 180 mg/dL

就寢時間   100–140 mg/dL

Hypoglycemia（低血糖）   低於 70 mg/dL

Hyperglycemia（高血糖）   高於 180 mg/dL

*根據 2009 年美國糖尿病協會臨床建議。你的糖尿病
醫療組也許會有各自1指標。

Chinese - Blood Sugar Levels & Target Numbers
Translation of this publication was supported by HRSA HCAP Grant
G92OA02204.
©2010 The Whittier Institute for Diabetes

PROJECT DULCE™
DIABETES EXCELLENCE ACROSS COMMUNITIES

8-11 詳閱食品標籤!

份量

標籤上的營養成分指的是「一份」。如果你打算吃超過一份，營養成分表中的含量就必須根據你吃下的份量調整。例如，如果份量是一杯而你打算吃下兩杯，營養成分標示的所有數字必須乘以二。

產品 － 原味優格

脂肪/膽固醇總數

依照低脂飲食，選擇每一份包含的脂肪不超過3公克的點心，燕麥片，乳製品，小菜，及低脂包裝肉品。肉類與起士的脂肪每一份不要超過65公克。

飽和及反式脂肪

飽和及反式脂肪會造成血中膽固醇含量增高。選擇脂肪中的飽和脂肪少於 1/3 及反式脂肪為零的食物。

鈉

依照低鈉飲食，選擇每天鈉的攝取量少於5%的食物，高於 20% 即為高鈉食物。

碳水化合物總數

要判定這份食物等於多少份碳水化合物，應該計算公克數。一份碳水化合物等於 15 公克的碳水化合物總數。

膳食纖維

每天至少攝取 25-35 公克的膳食纖維。如果有攝取 5 公克以上的膳食纖維，在計算碳水化合物的份量時可以從碳水化合物總數中扣除。

糖

每天攝取多少公克的糖已經計算成碳水化合物。不要用這個數字計算碳水化合物的份量。

維他命及礦物質

目標是每天攝取 100% 的維他命與礦物質。選擇各種食物而且不偏食才能達成此目標。

Nutrition Facts

Serving Size 1 Cup (248 g)
Servings Per Container 4

Amount Per Serving

Calories 150   Calories from Fat 35

	% Daily Value*
Total Fat 4 g	6%
Saturated Fat 2.5 g	12%
Trans Fat 0 g	
Cholesterol 20 mg	7%
Sodium 170 mg	7%
Total Carbohydrate 17 g	6%
Dietary Fiber 0 g	0%
Sugars 17 g	
Protein 13 g	

Vitamin A 4%	•	Vitamin C 6%	
Calcium 40%	•	Iron 0%	

*Percent Daily Values are based on a 2,000 calorie diet. Your daily values may be higher or lower depending on your calorie needs:

	Calories:	2,000	2,500
Total Fat	Less than	65 g	80 g
Sat Fat	Less than	20 g	25 g
Cholesterol	Less than	300 mg	300 mg
Sodium	Less than	2,400 mg	2,400 mg
Total Carbohydrate		300 g	375 g
Dietary Fiber		25 g	30 g

Calories per gram:
Fat 9 • Carbohydrate 4 • Protein 4

Chinese - Read The Food Label
Translation of this publication was supported by HRSA HCAP Grant # G92OA02204.
©2009 The Whittier Institute for Diabetes

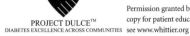

PROJECT DULCE™
DIABETES EXCELLENCE ACROSS COMMUNITIES

8–12 ABC về chăm sóc tiểu đường

Thử A1c, huyết áp, mỡ trong máu (Cholesterol)

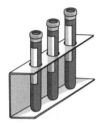

A1c = Glycosylated Hemoglobin, Glycohemoglobin (thử máu) có thể cho biết mức đường trung bình trong máu trong khoảng thời gian 2-3 tháng. Hội Tiểu Đường Hoa Kỳ khuyến cáo mức A1c dưới 7%.

Huyết Áp

Các con số trên (Tâm Trương) và các con số dưới (Tâm Thu) cho ta biết sức máu đẩy phía trong vách động mạch. Hội Tiểu Đường Hoa Kỳ khuyến cáo mức áp huyết phải dưới 130/80 mm/Hg.

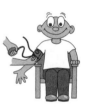

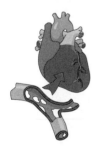

Mỡ trong máu (Cholesterol) =

nhóm hợp chất béo (Lipid Panel), Lipoprotein (thử máu) ADA khuyến cáo mức tổng số Cholesterol là < 200 mg/dL (LDL là <100 mg/dL), HDL trên 40 mg/dl ở nam giới và trên 50 mg/dl ở phụ nữ và triglycerides dưới 150 mg/dl.

Vietnamese - ABC's of Diabetes Management
Translation of this publication was supported by HRSA HCAP Grant # G92OA02204.
©2009 The Whittier Institute for Diabetes

PROJECT DULCE™
DIABETES EXCELLENCE ACROSS COMMUNITIES

8–13 Các Mức Đường Trong Máu Và Các Mục Tiêu Phải Đạt Tới

Tiền tiểu đường

100–125 mg/dL
A1c 5.7–6.4%

Định bệnh tiểu đường

126 mg/dL hoặc hơn
nhịn ăn cho 2 thử nghiệm khác nhau

hoặc

200 mg/dL hoặc hơn khi thử ngẫu nhiêr
có dấu hiệu tiểu đường

hoặc
A1c ≥ 6.5%

Các mục tiêu*

Nhịn ăn

70–130 mg/dL

2 giờ sau khi ăn miếng đầu tiên

Dưới 180 mg/dL

Khi đi ngủ

100–140 mg/dL

Mức đường thấp

Hypoglycemia (mức đường thấp)
Dưới 70 mg/dL

Mức đường cao

Hyperglycemia (mức đường cao)
Trên 180 mg/dL

Vietnamese - Blood Sugar Levels & Target Numbers
Translation of this publication was supported by HRSA HCAP Grant
G92OA02204.
©2010 The Whittier Institute for Diabetes

Permission granted by The Whittier Institute for Diabetes to
copy for patient education purposes. For additional information see
www.whittier.org

PROJECT DULCE™
DIABETES EXCELLENCE ACROSS COMMUNITIES

8–14 Đọc Nhãn Thực Phẩm!

Khẩu Phần (Serving Size)
Coi bao nhiêu khẩu phần trong hộp. Các dữ kiện dinh dưỡng nơi nhãn là cho từng "khẩu phần". Tất cả những con số ghi trên nhãn là các số lượng cho một khẩu phần. Nếu bạn ăn nhiều hơn là một khẩu phần, bạn cần điều chỉnh các con số theo khẩu phần chẳng hạn, nếu khẩu phần là 1 chén và bạn định ăn 2 chén, bạn cần nhân đôi số lượng ghi trên nhãn.

Sản Phẩm - Sữa Chua Thông Thường

Tổng số chất béo/Cholesterol
Để theo đuổi lối ăn ít chất béo, chọn cách ăn từng bữa nhỏ, ăn ngũ cốc (Cereal), thực phẩm có chất sữa, các món ăn nhỏ và thịt đóng gói có mỡ chừng 3 gram hay ít hơn cho mỗi khẩu phần. Thịt và phó-mát phải bằng hay ít mỡ hơn 5 gram cho mỗi khẩu phần.

Mỡ bão hòa và mỡ biến dạng (Saturated and Transfat).
Mỡ bão hòa và mỡ biến dạng có thể khiến mỡ trong máu (Blood Cholesterol) lên cao. Lựa các thực phẩm ít hơn 1/3 là mỡ bão hòa và không có mỡ biến dạng.

Muối (Sodium)
Để theo đuổi một lối ăn ít muối, lựa các thực phẩm có muối cỡ 5% hoặc ít hơn mức trị giá muối hang ngày. Nếu có mức muối từ 20% trở lên là mức cao về muối.

Tổng Hợp Đường và Tinh Bột (Carbohydrate)
Đây là con số gram để định xem thực phẩm có bao nhiêu khẩu phần tinh bột. Một khẩu phần có khoảng 15 grams tinh bột.

Chất Sợi (Dietary Fiber)
Nếu có 5 gram hoặc hơn về chất sợi thì có thể trừ đi từ số gram của tổng hợp nói trên khi tính khẩu phần tinh bột. Mỗi ngày nên có từ 20 tới 35 grams.

Đường
Số gram đường ghi trong nhãn đã được tính như một phần của tinh bột rồi. Đừng dùng con số này khi tính khẩu phần tinh bột.

Sinh Tố & Chất Khoáng
Mục tiêu là ăn đủ 100% mỗi chất hàng ngày. Ăn nhiều loại thực phẩm. Đừng nghĩ là một loại thực phẩm sẽ cho bạn đủ các chất trên.

Nutrition Facts

Serving Size 1 Cup (248 g)
Servings Per Container 4

Amount Per Serving

Calories 150	Calories from Fat 35

	% Daily Value*
Total Fat 4 g	**6%**
Saturated Fat 2.5 g	**12%**
Trans Fat 0 g	
Cholesterol 20 mg	**7%**
Sodium 170 mg	**7%**
Total Carbohydrate 17 g	**6%**
Dietary Fiber 0 g	**0%**
Sugars 17 g	
Protein 13 g	

Vitamin A 4%	•	Vitamin C 6%
Calcium 40%	•	Iron 0%

*Percent Daily Values are based on a 2,000 calorie diet. Your daily values may be higher or lower depending on your calorie needs:

	Calories:	2,000	2,500
Total Fat	Less than	65 g	80 g
Sat Fat	Less than	20 g	25 g
Cholesterol	Less than	300 mg	300 mg
Sodium	Less than	2,400 mg	2,400 mg
Total Carbohydrate		300 g	375 g
Dietary Fiber		25 g	30 g

Calories per gram:
Fat 9 • Carbohydrate 4 • Protein 4

Vietnamese - Read The Food Label
Translation of this publication was supported by HRSA HCAP Grant # G92OA02204.
©2009 The Whittier Institute for Diabetes

Permission granted by The Whittier Institute for Diabetes to copy for patient education purposes. For additional information see www.whittier.org

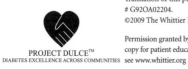

PROJECT DULCE™
DIABETES EXCELLENCE ACROSS COMMUNITIES

References

1. Centers for Disease Control and Prevention. *National Diabetes Fact Sheet.* 2007. Available at: http://www.cdc.gov/diabetes/pubs/pdf/ndfs_2007.pdf. Accessed October 28, 2009.

2. Harris MI, Flegal KM, Cowie CC, et al. Prevalence of diabetes, impaired fasting glucose, and impaired glucose tolerance in U.S. adults. The Third National Health and Nutrition Examination Survey, 1988–1994. *Diabetes Care.* 1998;21:518–524.

3. Babey SH, Brown ER, Chawla N, Diamant AL. *Diabetes in California: Findings from the 2001 California Health Interview Survey.* UCLA Center for Health Policy Research; 2003. Available at: https://www.policyarchive.org/handle/10207/8640. Accessed October 28, 2009.

4. Black S. Diabetes, diversity, and disparity: what do we do with the evidence? *Am J Public Health.* 2002;92:543–548.

5. Philis-Tsimikas A, Walker C, Rivard L, et al. Improvement in diabetes care of underinsured patients enrolled in Project Dulce. *Diabetes Care.* 2004;27:110–115.

6. Gilmer T, Walker C, Philis-Tsimikas A. Outcomes of Project Dulce: A culturally-specific diabetes management program. *Ann Pharmacother.* 2005;39:817–822.

7. Mazze RS, Etzwiler DD, Strock E, et al. Staged diabetes management. Toward an integrated model of diabetes care. *Diabetes Care.* 1994;17(suppl 1):56–66.

9 ▪ Psychosocial Care Related to Diabetes

A Chronic Disease

Having a chronic disease such as diabetes can be a challenge for the patient, the family and friends, as well as the healthcare professional. For the person with diabetes, every action—whether it's driving, eating, exercising, planning a vacation—circles around "how is this going to affect my diabetes?" "What do I need to do to stay safe and have healthy blood sugars?" "Will they let me on the airplane with my insulin and syringes?" A moment doesn't go by that the person with diabetes does not think about potential problems related to his or her diabetes management.

Frustration or a "why bother?" attitude may occur in healthcare professionals who feel like their medical recommendations are falling on deaf ears. "How many times do I have to tell you to exercise every day and stop drinking soda?" A very important message by Dr. Bill Polonsky and Dr. Susan Guzman was stated at a program for people with diabetes and the point was: "No one wants to be unhealthy or have negative things happen to them, but sometimes life gets in the way of us taking care of ourselves." Reflect on the patients that you see who may always be "out of control" or "noncompliant." Do they have personal challenges that are barriers to their own self-care?

The Office Visit: The Compliance Model versus the Empowerment Model

"I want you to walk for 45 minutes every day at a brisk pace and lose 15 pounds by the next visit!" The compliance model puts the healthcare professional at the center of care and fully responsible for making any health decisions. Think for a moment how you feel when someone tells you "You *have* to do *X*!" How motivated are you to do what was demanded of you? How do you feel when someone tells you what to do without asking for your input? Now imagine a different conversation in which someone using a nonjudgmental tone actually asks you, "Is there something you would be willing to do to feel better and improve your glucose levels?" This question places the choice solely on the patient's shoulders. The patient is at the center of care and fully responsible for making his or her health decisions. This gives the patient ownership of his or her choices and self-care.

According to Robert Anderson and Martha Funnel, the healthcare professional has four primary responsibilities to the patient with diabetes[1]:

1. Provide the diabetes expertise to develop an effective self-management plan
2. Educate the patient so that he or she can make an informed decision
3. Develop a collaborative relationship with the patient and significant others to be able to review and revise self-management plans as needed
4. Create a supportive environment for patients to make and maintain self-selected behavior changes

This is the patient empowerment approach philosophy[2]:

- Patient choices have the greatest effect on metabolic and other outcomes.
- Patients are in control of their self-management.
- The consequences related to self-management choices affect the patient directly, and therefore the patient should be the primary decision maker.

Table 9.1 shows an example of implementing the empowerment model.[2]

Table 9.1   Example of the Empowerment Model

DEFINE THE PROBLEM	IDENTIFY FEELINGS	IDENTIFY LONG-TERM GOALS	IDENTIFY SHORT-TERM GOALS	IMPLEMENT AND EVALUATE PLAN
"What is your greatest concern about diabetes?"	"How does this concern make you feel?"	"What would you like to see happen?" "What might get in the way of you dealing with this and how would you handle that?"	"Name one or two things you could do to improve this concern." "How are you going to get started?"	"Now that you have been working on this, how is it going?" "Is there anything you think you need to do differently?"
"What is your biggest challenge?"	"How does the challenge make you feel?"	"How important is it for you to overcome this challenge?" "Can you think of anything that might block you from moving forward to address this challenge?"	"List one or two things you could do to address this challenge." "Tell me what your plan is to get started."	"How did it go?" "Is there anything else you need to work on?"
Allows you to hear what is critical to the patient—the patient's greatest fear	Permits patient to acknowledge feelings. You may be the "neutral" person that they can be honest with	Identifies desired outcome, possible barriers, and commitment by patient	Facilitates a SMART goal: **S** specific **M** measurable **A** attainable **R** realistic **T** timely	Assesses whether the action plan is working or needs to be revised. Always acknowledge effort and provide nonjudgmental support

Factors in Behavior Change

You know that the recommendation for eating five to seven servings of fruits and vegetables a day and walking for 30 minutes is important, but do you do it *every day*? Knowledge does not translate to behavior change. In the Diabetes Attitudes, Wishes, and Needs Study (DAWN), reported rates of self-management behaviors were especially low for diet and exercise, with only 19.4% of people with type 1 and 16.2% of people with type 2 diabetes stating that they followed their providers' recommendations.[3]

At the time of diagnosis, more than 85% of patients report a high level of stress and feelings of shock, guilt, anger, anxiety, depression, and helplessness.[3] Emotional well-being is a huge factor in a patient's ability to make behavior changes. Consider the following points when you address behavior changes with your patients.

Patient Factors

- Belief that the benefits of therapy are worth the consequence
- Readiness to change
- Emotional well-being
- Memory, cognition, physical ability
- Communication skills, language
- Literacy and health literacy
- Confidence
- Skills
- Support systems
- Finances
- Access to healthy foods and a safe environment

Healthcare Team Factors

- Communication skills
- Quality of information
- Willingness to identify and address barriers
- Respectful, professional environment

- Regimen presented by team (if costly, difficult, or with many side effects, "compliance" diminishes)
- Avoid judgmental phrases such "good" or "bad" glucose

Remember, a behavior change is a cognitive and emotional process and it takes time. Patients are ultimately responsible for their own health care, but you have an opportunity to empower your patients by listening to them, asking them to identify areas they would like to improve, and helping them create a SMART goal (a goal that is specific, measurable, attainable, realistic, and timely). Evaluate the goal with the patient at each office visit and revise the goal as needed.

Depression

The World Health Organization projects depression will be the leading cause of disability and the second leading contributor to the global burden of disease by 2020.[4]

Diabetes is a 24-hour disease, and sometimes no matter how hard a person tries to manage the diabetes, glucose control is poor. This can be very frustrating. In the back of many people's mind is the fear of developing diabetes complications and premature death. People with diabetes not only have to deal with the daily rigors of diabetes self-care management issues, but they also face the same daily stresses that all of people experience regarding work, family, and finances. That is a lot to juggle for any person.

Studies find that the rate of depression is two or more times higher in people with diabetes.[5] The DAWN study, which looked at results from more than 5,000 people with diabetes, shows that after an average of 15 years from diagnosis many people still feared complications and felt a huge social and psychological burden related to caring for their diabetes. Forty-one percent reported poor well-being, but only 10% stated they received psychological treatment.[3] The chances of having depression can increase as a complication develops or there is some significant change in the patient's physical status.[6] Studies show depression leads to poorer physical and mental functioning, which affects diabetes self-management and increases the chance of an emergency room visit, hospitalization, or primary or specialty care visit.[7]

The following are signs and symptoms of depression. Not everyone who is depressed experiences every symptom. Often the symptoms last for weeks and may interfere with daily activities.

- Persistent sad, anxious, or "empty" mood
- Feelings of hopelessness, pessimism
- Persistent physical symptoms
- Restlessness, irritability
- Insomnia or change in sleeping habits (more sleep/less sleep)
- Feelings of worthlessness or guilt
- Thoughts of death or suicide or physical harm
- Appetite or weight changes
- Decreased energy, fatigue
- Difficulty concentrating, making decisions, or memory problems

Depression Screening Tools

A study in a primary care setting showed sensitivity and specificity of 97% and 67%, respectively, with patients not using psychotropic medications when asked the following questions[8]:

- During the past month, have you often been bothered by feeling down, depressed, or hopeless?
- During the past month, have you often been bothered by little interest or pleasure in doing things?

The Patient Health Questionnaire (PHQ-9) is a nine-question depression survey. The PHQ-9 is available in 31 languages at www.mapi-trust.org/services/questionnairelicensing/catalog-questionnaires. This survey asks patients to respond to nine short questions related to emotional health and asks them to rank how often they have experienced those feelings.

One of the important considerations when screening patients for depression is to have a concrete plan in place for referrals and follow-up care. Patients that are very depressed should be seen by a licensed clinician trained in that field of medicine.

Treatment Options

Medications[2]
- The selective serotonin reuptake inhibitor class is the most commonly prescribed group of antidepressants and includes fluoxetine, paroxetine, sertraline, citalopram, and escitalopram.
- Tricyclic antidepressants such as amitriptyline, desipramine, imipramine, nortriptyline, and doxepin.
- Other medications used for depression include venlafaxine, nefazodone, bupropion, mirtazapine, trazadone, and duloxetine.

Psychotherapy[2]
- Cognitive behavioral therapy emphasizes positive coping skills to work through any thoughts, behaviors, or feelings that may cause depression or negative thoughts.
- Interpersonal, family, client centered.

Exercise
- Studies by Otto, Trivedi, Church, and others show that burning off 350 calories three times a week while engaging in a sweat-inducing activity can reduce the symptoms of depression almost as much as an antidepressant can. Exercise was shown by brain imaging scans to stimulate the growth of neurons in certain areas of the brain that were damaged by depression.[9]

The Project Dulce + Improving Mood-Promoting Access to Collaborative Treatment (IMPACT) Study

The IMPACT study looked at 1,801 depressed older adults from 18 diverse primary care clinics across the United States for 2 years. Patients who received treatment had 116 less days of depression vs. the standard care group, lower healthcare costs, less physical pain, and a higher quality of life.[10]

Patients with diabetes from underserved and ethnic minority populations have higher rates of comorbid depression.[11] Project

Dulce, a program of Scripps Whittier Diabetes Institute, provides culturally appropriate diabetes nurse case management and self-management training that has been shown to improve diabetes outcomes among low-income, predominately Spanish speaking Latinos in San Diego County.

The Project Dulce + IMPACT study combined the current Project Dulce program and added a bilingual depression case manager to the Project Dulce team. Patients received the PHQ-9 depression screen, and those identified with clinically significant depression were referred to the depression care manager. The Project Dulce nurses, primary care provider, and the depression manager worked collaboratively with the patient. All patient materials were translated into Spanish at a low literacy level. Depression education blended traditional cultural beliefs and Western medicine. Out of the 499 patients screened for depression, 464 met the criteria to participate in the study. Sixty-five percent reported symptoms of depression for 2 years or more and 64% stated their family activities were negatively affected. Participants were more interested in receiving psychotherapy vs. pharmacotherapy. Financial stressors were noted as the most common cause of depression, followed by health concerns. At the end of the study PHQ-9 scores declined by an average of 7.5 points and diabetes self-care activities related to nutrition increased.

Culturally sensitive care is vital, especially in the area of mental health, where nuances of cultural beliefs and language can affect a patient's response to therapy.[10]

Resources for Psychosocial Care

African-American Family Services helps African American individuals, families, and communities reach a greater state of well-being through the delivery of community-based, culturally specific chemical health, mental health, and family preservation services:

2616 Nicollet Avenue, Minneapolis, MN 55408

Phone: 612-871-7878

Fax: 612-871-2811

Website: www.aafs.net

Anderson BJ, Rubin R. *Practical Psychology for Diabetes Clinicians: Effective Techniques for Key Behavioral Issues.* 2nd ed. Alexandria, VA: American Diabetes Association; 2003.

The Behavioral Diabetes Institute is a great resource for patients and healthcare professionals. A video archive contains professional education programs: www.behavioraldiabetes.org

IMPACT Evidenced-Based Depression Care: http://impact-uw.org

The MacArthur Initiative on Depression and Primary Care at Dartmouth and Duke: www.depression-primarycare.org/clinicians/toolkits/materials/

National Institute of Mental Health, results from the STAR*D trial: www.nimh.nih.gov/health/trials/practical/stard/index.shtml

National Suicide Prevention Lifeline 24-hr hotline: 1-800-273-8255 (TTY: 1-800-799-4889)

Project Dulce: www.scripps.org/services/diabetes/project-dulce

US Department of Health and Human Services Substance Abuse and Mental Health Services Administration provides comprehensive information about mental health services and resources for professionals and the public: http://mentalhealth.samhsa.gov

Diabetes Resource Toolkit

Patient Education

9–1 Depression and Diabetes

9–2 Diabetes: Your Emotional Response

9–3 Stress

9–1 DEPRESSION AND DIABETES

Do you . . .

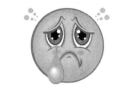

Feel Worried or Anxious

Have a Hard Time Concentrating

Forget Things

Get Headaches

Sleep Too Much or Not Enough

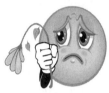

Feel Very Tired

Feel Sad or Empty

Feel Like You Don't Matter

Notice an Unplanned Weight Gain or Loss

There is help.

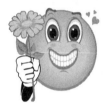

American Diabetes Association statistics show depression affects:

- 3–5% of general population
- 15–20% of people with diabetes

If you have any or a combination of these feelings, you may have symptoms of depression or stress.

- Please talk to your Doctor, Nurse, Social Worker, or any other Healthcare Professional.

Log on to Mental Health America for information: http://www.nmha.org/

9–2 DIABETES: YOUR EMOTIONAL RESPONSE

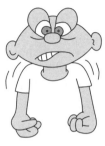

People react in different ways when they are told they have diabetes. Some are angry at their friends, family, or doctor. Others are sad and may cry periodically, for weeks or months. Others feel guilty, thinking that if they had not eaten certain foods, they would not have diabetes. Some refuse to believe they have diabetes. Many ask "why me?" These thoughts and feelings can lead to depression with feelings of despair and hopelessness. Remember that emotions affect blood glucose levels.

You may feel overwhelmed with all the new information you are receiving from your healthcare providers. This may be especially difficult for you to absorb when you are not feeling well. Remember to use this diabetes notebook for reference. We encourage you to call your diabetes educator at any time with questions or concerns.

Look to your family and friends for support. Let them know how you feel and let them share their feelings with you. Don't try to "protect" your family. The diabetes team encourages you to bring family members with you to your appointments—their lives are also affected by diabetes. Attending a diabetes support group can help you deal with your feelings. You can listen to and share experiences with others who know how it feels to have diabetes.

You will feel more in control of your diabetes as you learn how to make the necessary changes in your life. Making changes takes time and your diabetes team will work with you to help you achieve your goals. Remember, you are human and may relapse from time to time. Don't give up—just begin again the next day. You can feel good about making healthy lifestyle changes that include your entire family.

9–3 Stress

Introduction

Stress is a normal part of life, but one that can make it harder to control your blood glucose. There are several ways to fight stress and make your diabetes control easier.

What Is Stress?

Stress results when something causes your body to behave as if it were under attack. Sources of stress can be physical, like an injury or illness. Or they can be mental, like a problem in your marriage, job, health, or finances.

When stress occurs, the body gears up to take action. This preparation is called fight-or-flight response. In the fight-or-flight response, levels of many hormones shoot up. Their net effect is to make a lot of stored energy (glucose and fat) available to cells. These cells are then primed to help the body get away from danger.

In people who have diabetes, the fight-or-flight response does not work well. Insulin is not always able to let the extra energy into the cells, so glucose piles up in the blood.

Many sources of stress are chronic and continuous, making things worse. For example, it can take many months to recover from surgery. Stress hormones that are designed to deal with short-term danger stay turned on for a long time. As a result, long-term stress can cause long-term high glucose levels.

Many long-term sources of stress are mental. Your mind sometimes reacts to a nondangerous event as if it were a real threat. Like physical stress, mental stress can be short term—from taking a test to getting stuck in a traffic jam. It can also be long term—from working for a demanding boss to taking care of an aging parent. In mental stress, the body puts out hormones to no avail. Neither fighting nor fleeing is any help when the "enemy" is your own mind.

Scripps Whittier
Diabetes Institute

How Stress Affects Diabetes

In people who have diabetes, stress can alter blood glucose levels. It does this in two ways. First, people under stress may not take good care of themselves. They may drink more alcohol or exercise less. They may forget, or not have time, to test their glucose levels or plan good meals. Second, stress hormones may alter glucose levels directly.

References

1. Anderson BJ, Rubin RR. *Practical Psychology for Diabetes Clinicians: Effective Techniques for Key Behavioral Issues.* 2nd ed. Alexandria, VA: American Diabetes Association; 2002.

2. American Association of Diabetes Educators. *The Art and Science of Diabetes Self-Management Education: A Desk Reference for Healthcare Professionals.* Chicago, IL: American Association of Diabetes Educators; 2007.

3. Funnell MM. The Diabetes Attitudes, Wishes, and Needs Study. *Clin Diabetes.* 2006;24:154–155.

4. World Health Organization. Mental health and brain disorders: what is depression? Available at: http://www.who.int/mental_health/management/depression/definition/en/. Accessed November 17, 2009.

5. Peyrot M. Depression: a quiet killer by any name. *Diabetes Care.* 2003;26:2952–2953.

6. dLife. Diabetes and depression. Available at: http://www.dlife.com/dLife/do/ShowContent/daily_living/depression_and_coping. Accessed October 28, 2009.

7. Ciechanowski PS, Katon WJ, Russo JE. Depression and diabetes: impact of depressive symptoms on adherence, function and costs. *Arch Intern Med.* 2000;160:3278–3285.

8. Pomerantz JM. Screening for depression in primary care. *Medscape Today.* Available at: http://www.medscape.com/viewarticle/511167. Accessed October 28, 2009.

9. Kotz D. Depressed and coping: treating depression when medication fails. Available at: http://health.usnews.com/articles/health/brain-and-behavior/2009/04/24/depressed-treating-depression-drugs-medication-treatments-antidepressants.html. Accessed October 28, 2009.

10. IMPACT: evidence-based depression care. Available at: http://impact-uw.org/about. Accessed November 17, 2009.

11. Anderson D. Integrating depression care with diabetes care in real-world settings: lessons from the Robert Wood Johnson Foundation Diabetes Initiative. Available at: http://spectrum.diabetesjournals.org/content/20/1/10.full. Accessed October 28, 2009.

Index